Rebecca Diekmann

Nutritional State, Functionality & Mortality in Nursing Home Residents

Rebecca Diekmann

Nutritional State, Functionality & Mortality in Nursing Home Residents

- Results of a 12-month follow-up study

Südwestdeutscher Verlag für Hochschulschriften

Impressum/Imprint (nur für Deutschland/only for Germany)
Bibliografische Information der Deutschen Nationalbibliothek: Die Deutsche Nationalbibliothek verzeichnet diese Publikation in der Deutschen Nationalbibliografie; detaillierte bibliografische Daten sind im Internet über http://dnb.d-nb.de abrufbar.
Alle in diesem Buch genannten Marken und Produktnamen unterliegen warenzeichen-, marken- oder patentrechtlichem Schutz bzw. sind Warenzeichen oder eingetragene Warenzeichen der jeweiligen Inhaber. Die Wiedergabe von Marken, Produktnamen, Gebrauchsnamen, Handelsnamen, Warenbezeichnungen u.s.w. in diesem Werk berechtigt auch ohne besondere Kennzeichnung nicht zu der Annahme, dass solche Namen im Sinne der Warenzeichen- und Markenschutzgesetzgebung als frei zu betrachten wären und daher von jedermann benutzt werden dürften.

Verlag: Südwestdeutscher Verlag für Hochschulschriften GmbH & Co. KG
Dudweiler Landstr. 99, 66123 Saarbrücken, Deutschland
Telefon +49 681 37 20 271-1, Telefax +49 681 37 20 271-0
Email: info@svh-verlag.de

Zugl.: Bonn, Rheinische Friedrich-Wilhelms-Universität, Dissertation, 2011

Herstellung in Deutschland:
Schaltungsdienst Lange o.H.G., Berlin
Books on Demand GmbH, Norderstedt
Reha GmbH, Saarbrücken
Amazon Distribution GmbH, Leipzig
ISBN: 978-3-8381-2813-9

Imprint (only for USA, GB)
Bibliographic information published by the Deutsche Nationalbibliothek: The Deutsche Nationalbibliothek lists this publication in the Deutsche Nationalbibliografie; detailed bibliographic data are available in the Internet at http://dnb.d-nb.de.
Any brand names and product names mentioned in this book are subject to trademark, brand or patent protection and are trademarks or registered trademarks of their respective holders. The use of brand names, product names, common names, trade names, product descriptions etc. even without a particular marking in this works is in no way to be construed to mean that such names may be regarded as unrestricted in respect of trademark and brand protection legislation and could thus be used by anyone.

Publisher: Südwestdeutscher Verlag für Hochschulschriften GmbH & Co. KG
Dudweiler Landstr. 99, 66123 Saarbrücken, Germany
Phone +49 681 37 20 271-1, Fax +49 681 37 20 271-0
Email: info@svh-verlag.de

Printed in the U.S.A.
Printed in the U.K. by (see last page)
ISBN: 978-3-8381-2813-9

Copyright © 2011 by the author and Südwestdeutscher Verlag für Hochschulschriften GmbH & Co. KG and licensors
All rights reserved. Saarbrücken 2011

TABLE OF CONTENT

LIST OF TABLES		III
LIST OF FIGURES		IV
CHAPTER ONE		
	GENERAL INTRODUCTION	1
CHAPTER TWO		
	COMPARISON OF TWO DIFFERENT APPROACHES FOR THE APPLICATION OF THE MINI NUTRITIONAL ASSESSMENT IN NURSING HOMES: RESIDENT INTERVIEWS VERSUS ASSESSMENT BY NURSING STAFF	9
CHAPTER THREE		
	SPECIFIC BLOOD MARKERS OF NUTRITIONAL STATUS IN NURSING HOME RESIDENTS	29
CHAPTER FOUR		
	FUNCTIONALITY AND MORTALITY IN OBESE NURSING HOME RESIDENTS – AN EXAMPLE OF 'RISK FACTOR PARADOX'?	62
CHAPTER FIVE		
	GENERAL DISCUSSION	83

ABBREVIATIONS

ADL	Activities of Daily Living
AKE	Austrian Society for Clinical Nutrition
BIA	Bioimpedance analysis
BMI	Body mass index
CC	Calf circumference
CI	Confidence interval
DEXA	Dual X-Ray Absorptiometry
EDTA	Ethylenediaminetetraacetic acid
ELISA	Enzyme Linked Immunosorbent Assay
IQR	Interquartile range
f	Female
GDS	Geriatric Depression Scale
HGS	Handgrip strength
κ	Kappa index
kcal	Kilocalories
kg	Kilogram
m	Male
m^2	Square meter
MAC	Mid-arm circumference
MJ	Mega Joule
MMSE	Mini Mental State Examination
MNA	Mini Nutritional Assessment
MNAsf	MNA-Short Form
MUST	Malnutrition Universal Screening Tool
n	Number
n.s.	Not significant
NRS	Nutritional Risk Screening
SD	Standard deviation
PEG	Percutaneous endoscopic gastrostomy
PEM	Protein-Energy-Malnutrition
TUG	Timed 'up and go' test
WHO	World Health Organisation
y	Years

LIST OF TABLES

Table I: Characteristics of participants 15

Table II: Contingency table for MNAsf 17

Table III: Comparison of selected items of the MNA by resident interviews versus assessment by nursing staff 17

Table IV: Comparison of the MNA categorisation obtained by the two approaches ... 18

Table V: Six-month mortality rate in the three categories of the MNA – resident interviews 20

Table VI: Baseline characteristics of all participants I 36

Table VII: Baseline characteristics of all participants II 37

Table VIII: Baseline and follow-up characteristics of survivors 38

Table IX: Cut-off values and prevalence of low nutrient levels respectively nutrient deficiencies at t_0 40

Table X: Blood parameters in t_0 and t_{12} 42

Table XI: Comparison of blood level (non tube-fed vs. tube-fed) 43

Table XII: Nutrient status of deceased and survivors at t_0 44

Table XIII: Characteristics at baseline 68

Table XIV: BMI distribution of all participants, deceased and surviving participants ... 71

Table XV: Follow-up data of function stratified for BMI groups 72

LIST OF FIGURES

Figure I: Scatter plot of for the MNAsf: resident interview versus screening by nursing staff 16

Figure II: Scatter plot of the full MNA score resident vs. nursing staff..................... 19

Figure III: Prevalence of relevant chronic diseases in nursing home residents (t_0).. 39

Figure IV: Number of nutrient deficiencies at t_0 40

Figure V: Number of nutrient deficiencies per resident (t_0)..................................... 41

Figure VI: Box plots of nutrient levels of survivors at t_0 and t_{12} (n=121) 42

Figure VII: Prevalence of low blood levels (survivors vs. deceased) at t_0 44

Figure VIII: Survival (cum.) in the vitamin D groups (t_0).. 45

Figure IX: Prevalence of diseases stratified for BMI groups..................................... 70

Figure X: Kaplan-Meier survival estimated by BMI categories 71

CHAPTER ONE

General Introduction

A poor nutritional status due to an insufficient intake of energy, macro- and/or micronutrients (general and/or specific malnutrition) is a well-known independent risk factor for enhanced functional decline as well as for increased morbidity and mortality rates in elderly people (MORLEY AND SILVER 1995, BAUER ET AL. 2006); moreover, malnutrition is a decisive factor for an early nursing home admission (KWON ET AL 2007, SHARKEY ET AL. 2006, VISSER ET AL. 2006, BISCHOFF-FERRARI ET AL. 2004, STANGA ET AL 2004, VOLPATO ET AL. 2004, AMARANTOS ET AL. 2001, ZULIANI ET AL. 2001).

A low nutritional intake in the elderly is the consequence of a variety of different circumstances which often appear in combination (PIRLICH AND LOCHS 2001): low physical activity, pain, tremor, dry mouth, swallowing or chewing difficulties, smell or taste failures, dementia, depression, social isolation, financial problems and others. Age-associated changes in the complex system of regulating nutritional intake comprising enteral, neuronal and endocrine mechanisms lead to a decline in hunger and appetite, and an increased sensation of satiety (BAUER ET AL. 2008, DE CASTRO 1993). The change of hormone levels decisively influences the nutritional status and the food intake (BAUER ET AL. 2007, STURM ET AL. 2003, MACINTOSH ET AL. 1999, MORLEY 1997). Multimorbid seniors often receive multimedication which further decreases nutritional intake due to adverse effects such as chronic nausea, dry mouth, anorexia, etc. The inadequate intake of energy and nutrients is leading to a dramatic loss in muscle mass (sarcopenia), fat mass and nutrient reserves decreasing the ability to overcome acute illness (BAUER ET AL. 2006).

The prevalence of malnourished elderly has been evaluated in numerous studies (GASKILL ET AL. 2008, SALVI ET AL. 2008, PAULY ET AL. 2007, PIRLICH ET AL. 2006). Obviously, the prevalence of general malnutrition depends on the setting (outpatients, homebound, hospitalised or institutionalised individuals) and the assessment method used and ranged between 5% and 85% (PAULY ET AL. 2007, STANGA 2004). Only few and inconsistent information is available with respect to the micronutrient status (VOLKERT ET AL. 1992, VELLAS ET AL. 2000, RAFFOUL ET AL. 2006): generally low plasma values were, however, reported for vitamin C and vitamin D. Since the need for micronutrients remains constant or is even increased in pathophysiological situations whereas the energy requirements decline with age, an adequate intake of minerals and vitamins requires the preferential consumption of nutrient dense food (DGE 2007, DACH 2000).

Our knowledge with respect to the nutritional situations of nursing home residents is still scarce. In a current study it was shown that one third of German elderly female nursing home residents who were able to eat without any help had an energy intake of less than 1700 kcal/d; dependent residents had an even lower average intake of only 1130 kcal/d (SCHMID ET AL. 2003). In an Australian nursing home, an inadequate energy intake was found in 60% of the residents (GRIEGER AND NOWSON 2007). With regard to protein status, a proportion of approximately 30% newly admitted nursing home residents in Sweden are suffering from protein-energy-malnutrition (PEM). This share increased up to more than 40% in residents released from acute hospital care (CHRISTENSSON ET AL. 1999). It has been demonstrated that a reduced protein and/or energy intake (protein/energy malnutrition) is related to frailty, a geriatric syndrome with multifactorial origin and prevalence up to 27% in the population aged 65 years and older (KAISER ET AL. 2009). In a national cross-sectional study recently performed in 10 German nursing homes (773 residents), 8% of males and 6% of females had a dramatic low BMI (<18.5). Using the Mini Nutritional Assessment 11% of residents were classified malnourished. Interestingly, still 20% of men and 21% of women were obese (BMI $\geq$30) (HESEKER AND STEHLE 2008). Comparable results were obtained in a recent study assessing newly admitted nursing home residents: the prevalence of obesity increased from 15% to more than 25% in the years from 1992 to 2002 (LAPANE AND RESNIK 2005). In which way overweight/obesity is influencing life quality, functionality and morbidity in older residents is not known.
The few studies focusing on the nutritional status, indicated by blood nutrients, showed inconsistent results. In a population of both nursing home residents and community-dwelling elderly, it was shown that vitamin C and niacin levels were acceptable whereas deficits in vitamin A, thiamine and riboflavin were obvious (HARRILL AND CERVONE 1977). Loewik and co-workers observed a significant lower mean level of several vitamins in Dutch nursing home residents in comparison to free

and more independently living elderly (LOEWIK ET AL. 1992). With regard to vitamin D, a highly prevalent deficiency was shown worldwide (HOLICK 2007). In German nursing home residents, the intake (3-day protocol) of the micronutrients (except vitamin A and niacin) analyzed were clearly below the reference values (DACH 2000). Both, vitamin and fibre, did not reach 50% of the recommendation (HESEKER AND STEHLE 2008). Scientific work focusing on the nutritional status of nursing home residents is hampered by various factors. Due to a high prevalence of cognitively impaired residents, one-on-one interviews are generally not applicable; consequently, assessment has to be performed by the nursing staff. This affords corresponding competence of the staff. Furthermore, it is still questionable which screening and/or assessment method provides reliable results and should, thus, be used in routine work. Evaluation of blood analysis requires the availability of reference values. Presently, we use data published for healthy adults. Finally, the "optimal" body weight for morbid elderly is not defined yet.

References I

AMARANTOS E, MARTINEZ A, DWYER J. Nutrition and Quality of Life in Older Adults. *J Gerontol. 2001,56A:54-64.*

BAUER JM, VOLKERT D, WIRTH R, VELLAS B, THOMAS D, KONDRUP J, PIRLICH M, WERNER H, SIEBER CC. Diagnosing malnutrition in the elderly. *Dtsch Med Wochenschr. 2006;131:223-227.*

BAUER JM, WIRTH R, TROEGNER J, ERDMANN J, EBERL T, HEPPNER HJ, SCHUSDZIARRA V, SIEBER CC. Ghrelin, anthropometry and nutritional assessment in geriatric hospital patients. *Z Gerontol Geriatr. 2007;40:31–36*

BAUER JM, WIRTH R, VOLKERT D, WERNER H, SIEBER CC. Malnutrition, Sarkopenie und Kachexie im Alter – Von der Pathophysiologie zur Therapie. *Dtsch Med Wochenschr. 2008;133:305-310.*

BISCHOFF-FERRARI HA, DIETRICH T, ORAV EJ, HU FB, ZHANG Y, KARLSON EW, DAWSON HUGHES B. Higher 25-hydroxyvitamin D concentrations are associated with better lower-extremity function in both active and inactive persons aged $\geq$ 60 y. *Am J Clin Nutr. 2004;80:752-8.*

CHRISTENSSON L, UNOSSON M, EK AC. Malnutrition in elderly people newly admitted to a community resident home. *J Nutr Health Aging 1999;3(3):133-9.*

DACH Referenzwerte Deutsche Gesellschaft für Ernährung, Österreichische Gesellschaft für Ernährung, Schweizerische Gesellschaft für Ernährungsforschung, Schweizerische Vereinigung für Ernährung. Referenzwerte für die Nährstoffzufuhr. 1. Auflage. Umschau/ Braus-Verlag, Frankfurt/Main, 2000.

DE CASTRO JM. Age-related changes in spontaneous Food intake and Hunger in Humans. *Appetite 1993;21:255-272.*

DGE (DEUTSCHE GESELLSCHAFT FÜR ERNÄHRUNG) 2007. Internet-source: *http://www.dge-medienservice.de/editor/File/PDF/Essen-und-Trinken-im-Alter.pdf. 07/2010.*

GASKILL D, BLACK LJ, ISENRING EA, HASSALL S, SANDERS F, BAUER JD. Malnutrition prevalence and nutrition issues in residential aged care facilities. *Australas J Ageing. 2008;27(4):189-94.*

GRIEGER JA, NOWSON CA. Nutrition intake and plate waste from an Australian residential care facility. *Eur J Clin Nutr. 2007;61:655-663.*

HARRILL I, CERVONE N. Vitamin status of older women. *Am J Clin Nutr. 1977;30:431-440.*

HESEKER H, STEHLE P. Ernährung älterer Menschen in stationären Einrichtungen (ErnSTES-Studie). In: Deutsche Gesellschaft für Ernährung (Hrsg.): *Ernährungsbericht 2008. Druck: DCM – Druck Center Meckenheim GmbH – Meckenheim 2008;157-204.*

HOLICK MF. Vitamin D Deficiency. *N Engl J Med. 2007;357:266-281.*

KAISER MJ, BANDINELLI S, LUNENFELD B. The nutritional pattern of frailty – Proceedings from the 5th Italian Congress of Endocrinology of Aging, Parma, Italy, 27-28 March 2009. *Aging Male 2009;12(4):87-94.*

KWON J, SUZUKI T, KIM H, YISHIDA Y, IWASA H. Concomitant lower serum albumin and vitamin D levels are associated with decreased objective physical performance among Japanese community-dwelling elderly. *Gerontol. 2007;53:322-328.*

LAPANE KL, RESNIK L. Obesity in nursing homes: An escalating problem. *J Am Geriatr Soc. 2005;53:1386-1391.*

LOEWIK MR, VAN DEN BERG H, SCHRIJVER J, ODINK J, WEDEL M, VAN HOUTEN P. Marginal nutritional status among institutionalized elderly women as compared to those living more independently (Dutch Nutrition Surveillance System). *J Am Coll Nutr. 1992;11(6):673-681.*

MACINTOSH CG, ANDREWS JM, JONES KL, WISHART JM; MORRIS HA, JANSEN JBMJ, MORLEY J, HOROWITZ M, CHAPMANN IM. Effects of age on concentrations of plasma cholecystokinin, glucagon-like peptide 1, and peptide YY and their relation to appetite and pyloric motility. *Am J Clin Nutr. 1999;69:999–1006*

MORLEY JE. Anorexia of aging: physiologic and pathologic. *Am J Clin Nutr 1997;66:760-773.*

MORLEY, JE, SILVER AJ. Nutritional Issues in Nursing Home Care. *Ann Intern Med. 1995;123:850-859.*

PAULY L, STEHLE P, VOLKERT D. Nutritional situation of elderly nursing home residents. *Z Gerontol Geriatr. 2007;40:3–12.*

PIRLICH M, LOCHS H. Nutrition in the elderly. Best practice & Research Clinical *Gastroenterology 2001;15(6):869-884.*

PIRLICH M, SCHÜTZ T, NORMAN K, GASTELL S, LÜBKE HJ, BISCHOFF SC, BOLDER U, FRIELING T, GÜLDENZOPH H, HAHN K, JAUCH KW, SCHINDLER K, STEIN J, VOLKERT

D, WEIMANN A, WERNER H, WOLF C, ZÜRCHER G, BAUER P, LOCHS H. The German hospital malnutrition study. *Clin Nutr. 2006;25(4):563-72.*

RAFFOUL W, FAR MS, CAYEUX M-C, BERGER MM. Nutritional status and food intake in nine patients with chronic low-limb ulcers and pressure ulcers: importance of oral supplements. *Nutrition 2006;22:82-88.*

SALVI F, GIORGI R, GRILLI A, MORICHI V, ESPINOSA E, SPAZZAFUMO L, MARINOZZI ML, DESSÌ-FULGHERI P. Mini Nutritional Assessment (short form) and functional decline in older patients admitted to an acute medical ward. *Aging Clin Exp Res. 2008;20(4):322-8*

SCHMID A, WEISS M, HESEKER H. Recording the nutrient intake of nursing home residents by food weighing method and measuring the physical activity. *J Nutr Health Aging 2003;7(5):294-5.*

SHARKEY JR, ORY MG, BRANCH LG. Severe Elder Obesity and 1-Year Diminished Lower Extremity Physical Performance in Homebound Older Adults. *J Am Geriatr Soc. 2006;54:1407-1413.*

STANGA Z, ALLISON S, VANDWOUDE M. Nutrition in the elderly. In: *Basics in Clinical Nutrition 3rd edition, Galen, ESPEN 2004.*

STURM K, MACINTOSH CG, PARKER BA, WISHART J,HOROWITZ M, CHAPMAN IM. Appetite, Food Intake, and Plasma Concentrations of Cholecystokinin, Ghrelin, and Other Gastrointestinal Hormones in Undernourished Older Women and Well-Nourished Young and Older Women. *J Clin Endocrinol Metab. 2003;88(8):3747–3755.*

VELLAS B, GUIGOZ Y, BAUMGARTNER M, GARRY PJ, LAUQUE S, ALBAREDE JL. Relationship between nutritional markers and the mini-nutritional assessment in 155 older persons. *J Am Geriatr Soc. 2000;48(10):1300-1309.*

VISSER M, DEEG DJH, PUTS MTE, SEIDELL JC, LIPS P. Low serum concentrations of 25-hydroxyvitamin D in older persons and the risk of nursing home admission. *Am J Clin Nutr. 2006;84:616-622.*

VOLKERT D, FRAUENRATH C, MICOL W, KRUSE W, OSTER P, SCHLIERF G. Nutritionnal status of the very old: anthropometric and biochemical findings in apparently healthy women in old people's homes. *Aging (Milano) 1992:4(1):21-28.*

VOLPATO S, ROMAGNONI F, SOATTIN L, BLÈ A, LEOCI V, BOLLINI, C, FELLIN R, ZULIANI G. Body Mass Index, Body Cell mass, and 4-Year All-Cause Mortality Risk in Older Nursing Home Residents. *J Am Geriatr Soc. 2004;52:886-891.*

ZULIANI G, ROMAGNONI F, VOLPATO S, SOATTIN L, LEOCI V, BOLLINI MC, BUTTARELLO M, LOTTO D, FELLIN R. Nutritional Parameters, Body Composition, and Progression of Disability in Older Disabled Residents Living in Nursing Homes. *J Gerontol. 2001;56A(4):212-216.*

AIMS OF THE THESIS

The purpose of this follow-up study in a population of nursing home residents was to further improve our knowledge with respect to the assessment and evaluation of the nutritional status. In this regard, the following questions should be answered:

- CHAPTER TWO:
  Is the screening tool Mini Nutritional Assessement (MNA) performed by one-on-one interview with the nursing home residents themselves or by assessment with the help of the according nursing staff a reliable and practicable method to screen the nutritional status of nursing home residents? Does the tool provide a predictive value?

- CHAPTER THREE:
  How is the nutrient status regarding specific blood markers in the population of nursing home residents and how influence these blood levels the functionality and morbidity in the observed population?

- CHAPTER FOUR:
  In which way is obesity, defined as BMI above 30 kg/m^2, influencing functional abilities and mortality of nursing home residents?

CHAPTER TWO

Comparison of two different approaches for the application of the Mini Nutritional Assessment in nursing homes: resident interviews versus assessment by nursing staff

Kaiser et al, published in J Nutr Health Aging 2009;13(10):863-9.

Abstract

Background: When the Mini Nutritional Assessment (MNA®) was developed, the authors did not specifically focus on the nursing home setting. Due to a number of particularities of nursing home residents, such as cognitive and linguistic disabilities, a number of uncertainties with regard to its application await clarification. **Aims and objectives:** The aim of this study was to compare the results of two different modes of MNA application in nursing homes: resident interviews versus assessment by nursing staff. **Method:** The MNA was applied to 200 residents of two municipal nursing homes in Nuremberg, Germany. First one-on-one interviews of the residents were conducted by two researchers from our group. Next, the MNA was applied by the attending nursing staff, who were blinded to the results of the first MNA. To evaluate the prognostic properties of the two different approaches, data on mortality of the screened residents were collected during a six-month follow-up period. **Results:** Among 200 residents (f 147 m 53, f 86.5±7.4 y. m 83.0±8.5 y.), the MNA could be applied to 138 residents (69.0%) by one-on-one interviews and to 188 residents (94.0%) by the nursing staff. 15.2% of the residents were categorised as malnourished by the interviews and 8.7% by the nursing staff's assessment (n=138). The agreement of the two forms was low for the short form (weighted κ=0.31; 95% CI: 0.14 - 0.47) as well as for the full MNA (weighted κ=0.35; 95% CI: 0.27 - 0.44). After exclusion of residents with cognitive impairment (n=89), agreement for the full version increased (weighted κ=0.47, 95% CI 0.25 - 0.68). 25 (12.5%) study participants deceased during the follow-up period. Mortality was significantly associated with the MNA categories for both approaches, while the MNA application by the nursing staff proved to be superior (nursing staff p<0.001, residents p<0.05). **Conclusions:** The results of the MNA in nursing home residents may differ substantially when resident interviews are compared to assessment by nursing staff. The authors recommend that the MNA should be routinely applied by the nursing staff as thus application rate is higher and interference with cognitive as well as linguistic deficits is lower. In future studies, the mode of MNA application in nursing home residents should be clearly stated to facilitate comparability of results.

Key words: Nutritional screening, Mini Nutritional Assessment, malnutrition, nursing home.

Introduction

Malnutrition has been identified as a frequent problem among the frail elderly in most industrialized countries. It is associated with loss of functionality, lower quality of life, higher risk of morbidity and increased mortality (1-4,7). The highest prevalence rates for malnutrition were reported for elderly patients in hospitals and those living in nursing homes, with a range of between 5% and 70%, depending on the definition of malnutrition applied (5,6). Still, no gold standard exists for the latter. In 2003, the European Society for Clinical Nutrition and Metabolism (ESPEN) recommended three nutritional screening tools to be applied according to the population which is to be screened (4). These tools were the Malnutrition Universal Screening Tool (MUST), the Nutritional Risk Screening (NRS) and the Mini Nutritional Assessment (MNA). The latter has been regarded as the most suitable screening tool for the geriatric population. The original study, published in 1994 by Guigoz, Vellas and Garry, was based on three different cohorts of elderly persons from the Toulouse area and from the New Mexico Aging Progress Study (8,9). The MNA was developed for practicable and rapid nutritional screening in frail elderly people. It was designed to be completed in 10 to 15 minutes, with the intention of targeting early nutritional intervention (10). Meanwhile, the MNA has become the best documented screening tool for malnutrition in the elderly, with more than 10,000 study participants in different settings (6).

With regard to its application in nursing homes, several studies have been published over the last two years (11-19). However, the application of the MNA may be hampered by cognitive and linguistic disabilities, which are frequently present among nursing home residents. Similar problems have been described in an application study among hospitalized geriatric patients (20). Under these circumstances, the MNA was completed by the attending nurses in most cases. Potential differences between these two approaches of MNA application – one-on-one resident interview versus assessment by nursing staff – have not been systematically analyzed before for only Tsai et al. published a comparison with caregivers` assessment, focusing exclusively on the two MNA questions that are exploring self-assessment with regard to nutritional status and general health (11). In the present study, we analyzed these two approaches for the short form and the full MNA. We also tested their prognostic value with regard to mortality in a six-month follow-up period.

Subjects

Two hundred residents from two municipal nursing homes in Nuremberg, Germany, were recruited for this study from June to December 2007. Residents were excluded if they were under 65 years of age, terminally ill or did not give informed consent (resident or legal proxy, respectively). The study protocol was approved by the ethics committees of the Friedrich-Alexander-University of Erlangen-Nuremberg, Germany, and the Rheinische Friedrich-Wilhelms-University of Bonn, Germany.

Method

A nutrition scientist (Kaiser R - KR) and a physician (Winning K - WK) approached all residents in the two Nuremberg nursing homes and/or their legal proxy. After obtaining informed consent, all participants were examined in an identical manner. First, the MNA was completed with the help of the resident in a one-on-one interview, conducted by either WK or KR. Afterwards, the MNA for each subject was completed by the attending nursing staff member, who was blinded with regard to the result of the initial MNA. Here all results with the exception of the sub-items F, Q and R (see below) were based on the estimation by the nursing staff, their experience and their awareness of the medical records. In six cases the length of stay was less than three months (one month in two cases, two months in four cases); here the nursing staff members completed the MNA with the knowledge and data available to them by that time. The two MNAs for each resident were always completed within one week.

The MNA consists of two parts: the MNA-Short Form (MNAsf) with six items (items A-G) and the full MNA which comprises the MNAsf and twelve additional items. The MNAsf was developed by Rubenstein in 2001 (27) and scores a maximum of 14 points. The screened subject is classified as "normal" with scores of 12 or more; below 12, the subject is "at risk of malnutrition". The full MNA (items G-R) contains 12 additional questions on their living situation, drug intake, skin lesions, anthropometric parameters, dietary and subjective assessment. The nutritional status is classified into three categories: 24 - 30 points indicate that the subject is well-nourished, 17 - 23.5 points indicate that the resident is at risk of malnutrition and up to 16.5 points mean that he/she is malnourished. In the present study, items F (BMI), Q (mid-arm circumference) and R (calf circumference) were assessed by KR and WK for both modes. The question about the residents' living situation (item G) always scored 0 points, due to the nursing home setting of the study. Cognitive status was determined by the Mini Mental State Examination by Folstein (MMSE) (21). The emotional status was tested by the short form of the Geriatric Depression Scale, validated by Lesher and Berryhill in 1994 (22). Anthropometric measurements were weight, knee height, mid-arm circumference (MAC) and calf circumference (CC). The measurements of all subjects were performed by the nutrition scientist (KR). The weight was measured to the nearest 0.1 kg using a weigh chair (type Arjo CFA 2000). The knee height was measured by a knee height sliding calliper provided by the Austrian Society for Clinical Nutrition (AKE) (23) in a sitting position. Bedridden residents were measured in a supine position. The knee and the ankle had to be bent at 90°. The knee height was recorded to the nearest 0.1 cm for all participants. The measurement was carried out as described by Chumlea (24). The body height was calculated using the equations developed by Chumlea et al. in a cohort beyond the age of 60 (25):

white non-Hispanic male: $78.31 + (1.94 \times \text{knee height}) - (0.14 \times \text{age})$

white non-Hispanic female: $82.21 + (1.85 \times \text{knee height}) - (0.21 \times \text{age})$

The Body Mass Index (BMI) was calculated by body weight (kg) divided by squared body height (m^2).

The measurements of the MAC and the CC were carried out with a flexible measuring tape and were recorded to the nearest 0.1 cm. The MAC was measured at the mid-point between the tip of the shoulder and the tip of the elbow between olecranon process and the acromion on the left side. The CC was measured at the widest point of the calf muscle without compressing the subcutaneous tissue of the patient in a supine or sitting position on the left side. The mean was taken from two consecutive measurements. Individual variables, such as gender, age, social and medical data, were collected from the medical records of the nursing home or from the nursing staff by way of a questionnaire. The Barthel's Index, developed in 1965 by Mahoney and Barthel (ADL) (26), was carried out by the nursing staff. Maximum score was 100 points; a score of >64 points was regarded as independent in activities of daily living, 35 – 64 points was indicative of being in need of assistance, while a score <35 points indicated need of care. During a six-month follow-up period, data on the residents' mortality were collected.

Statistics

Statistical analysis was performed using SPSS© version 16.0 (SPSS for windows, SPSS Inc., Chicago, IL, USA) and SAS (version 9.1, SAS Institute, Cary, NC, USA). Inter-rater reliability - in this context meaning the agreement between one-on-one interviews and assessment by nursing staff - was quantified by Cohen's kappa index (28) for the classified MNA outcome and the individual items of the long version of the MNA. In the case of ordinal items with more than two levels, the weighted kappa value was estimated. To examine whether differences between the two ratings depart from chance variation, i.e. whether there are systematic differences between the two assessments, the McNemar and the Bowker test for symmetry was used, as appropriate. Correlation between MNA score values was quantified with the Spearman rank correlation coefficient. Statistical significant differences were taken by a p-values < 0.05.

Results

Study population

Out of 322 residents living in the two nursing homes, 122 persons (98 females and 24 males) were not eligible for the present study. For 42 residents, their proxies did not agree in their participation (34.4% of non-participating residents). Proxies could not be contacted in another 14 cases (11.5%). 28 residents were personally unwilling to participate in the study (23.0%). Ten residents were terminally ill (8.2%) and 10 residents were under age 65 (8.2%). Other residents did not participate for various reasons such as acute hospitalisation, infection with multi-resistant bacterial strains, etc. (18 residents, 14.8%). The mean age of the non-participating residents (82.8±11.5 years) was significantly lower than that of the participating residents.

Of the 200 residents included, 147 were female and 53 male (mean age 85.5±7.8 years). All participants were Caucasians. Women were significantly older than men (p<0.05). The majority of included residents were multimorbid, with diabetes mellitus being present in 36.0% of the residents, arterial hypertension in 76.5%, chronic heart failure in 74.0%, residual symptoms after cerebral ischemia in 29.0%, and osteoarthritis in 31.0%. The mean number of drugs taken on a daily basis was 7.8±4.9 (range 0-24). The GDS was completed in 71.0% of the residents. 50.0% of these were found to have a score indicative of overt depression. The MMSE was applicable to 91.0% of the residents. 75.5 % of theses showed results indicating relevant cognitive impairment (<25 points). With regard to the activities of daily living (ADL), 28.0% of the residents were independent and 29.5% needed assistance. 42.5% required a high level of care. The characteristics and anthropometric data of the participants are shown in table I.

Table I: Characteristics of participants

	Women	Men
Number of participants	147	53
Age [y]*	86.5 (± 7.4)°	83.0 (± 8.5)°
ADL [points/100]	40 [15-65]⁺	45 [20-67.5]⁺
GDS [points/15]	5 [3-8]⁺	4 [2-8.5]⁺
MMSE [points/30]	19 [1-24.5]⁺	19 [7.5-29]⁺
Body weight [kg]*	63.2 (± 13.9)°	74.6 (± 15.5)°
BMI [kg/m^2]	26.5 (± 5.5)°	25.6 (± 4.4)°
MAC [cm]	28.3 (± 4.5)°	29.1 (± 4.5)°
CC [cm]	32.6 (± 5.2)°	33.0 (± 4.3)°

⁺median (1.quartile-3. quartile), °mean ± SD, * (t-test p<0.05)
ADL = Activities of Daily Living, GDS = Geriatric Depression Scale,
MMSE = Mini Mental State Examination, MAC = Mid-arm circumference,
CC = calf circumference⁺

Application of the MNA

Application of the MNA by one-on-one interview of the resident was possible in 69.0% (n=138). The reasons for non-applicability included communicative deficits, such as aphasia and cognitive impairment in 25%, tube feeding in 5% and amputation of both lower limbs in 1%, as CC could not be measured in these cases. The MNA could be completed by assessment of the nursing staff in 94.0% of the cases (n=188). Again, the MNA could not be applied due to tube feeding (5%) or lower limb amputations (1%). The following analyses are based on the subset of data that included only those residents for whom the MNA was completed by both approaches (n=138).

MNA short form (MNAsf)

Figure I shows a scatter plot of score points obtained by the MNAsf for resident interviews versus assessment by nursing staff. The size of bubbles indicates the frequency when scoring results of both approaches met. The cut-offs of the two categories of the MNAsf – "normal" and "at risk of malnutrition" - are represented by horizontal and vertical lines.

Figure I: Scatter plot of for the MNAsf: resident interview versus screening by nursing staff

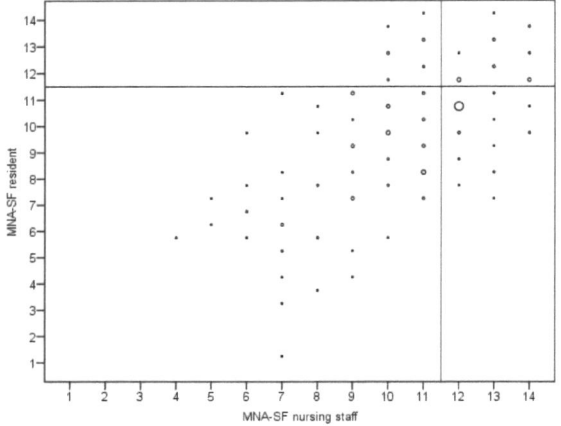

The size of the bubbles indicates the frequency when scoring results of both approaches met. The cut-offs of the two categories of the MNAsf are represented by the horizontal and vertical lines.

According to the one-on-one interviews 76.1% of residents were categorised as "at risk of malnutrition", while 63.8% were categorised in the same group by the nursing staff, respectively (table II). So, a higher number of residents was categorised as "normal" when they were screened by the nursing staff. Correlation between the two modes of application was moderate (Spearman rank correlation coefficient 0.60, $p<0.001$). The test of symmetry revealed a significant difference ($p<0.05$, McNemar test). Agreement was only fair (kappa 0.31; 95% CI: 0.14 - 0.47). In addition, we analyzed five sub-items of the MNAsf separately to identify the most obvious differences between the two approaches (table III). With regard to item A, which addresses loss of appetite and reduced food intake, it was noticed that 14 residents reported severe loss of appetite, while only six residents were placed in this category by the nursing staff. Agreement between the two approaches was only low for this item. When confronted with the second question of the MNAsf that explores 'weight loss during the last three months' residents choose the option 'does not know' in 23.0%, while the nursing staff provided a definitive answer in every case. There was also a considerable discrepancy with regard to the option 'no weight loss' (57.9%

resident vs. 78.2% nursing staff). Item C mobility showed the highest agreement among the items of the short form (weighted kappa 0.52). For this item, no significant difference was found between the two approaches. With regard to item D, 29.8% of the residents indicated that they suffered from acute disease or psychological stress in the past three months, which is close to the 28.9% determined by the nursing staff's assessment, but again, agreement was only fair ($\kappa=0.28$). For item E the rating of presence of depression and dementia significantly skewed ($p<0.05$) the way that residents estimated their neuropsychological problems as less severe than the nursing staff did. Anyhow, between the two approaches a fair but significant agreement (weighted $\kappa=0.19$) was observed.

Table II: Contingency table for MNAsf

			Nursing staff		
			Well-nourished	Risk of malnutrition	Total
Resident interviews	Well-nourished	n	21	12	33
	Risk of malnutrition	n	29	76	105
	Total	n	50	88	138

Table III: Comparison of selected items of the MNA by resident interviews versus assessment by nursing staff

	(weighted)§ kappa (95% CI)	Bowker (McNemar)$^\$$ test of symmetry (difference)
A Anorexia	§0.12 (0-0.25)	$p<0.001$
B Weight loss	§0.19 (0.07-0.32)	$p<0.001$
C Mobility	§0.52 (0.40-0.63)	n.s.
D Acute disease	0.28 (0.11-0.46)	$^\$$n.s.
E Neuropsychological problems	§0.19 (0.06-0.32)	$p<0.05$
O Nutritional status	§0.03 (0-0.18)	n.s.
P Health status	§0.03 (0-0.14)	n.s.

n.s. = not significant

Full MNA

Resident interviews yielded a mean score of 21.4 points (median 22, Interquartile range [IQR] 19 - 24.5). 15.2% of the residents were categorised as malnourished, 52.9% as being at risk of malnutrition and 31.9% as being well-nourished. For the same residents, based on the assessment by the nursing staff, the mean score of the total MNA was 21.3 points (median 22, IQR 18.5 - 24). 8.7% were categorised as malnourished, 54.3% as being at risk of malnutrition and 37.0% as being well-nourished. The correlation between the two scores was moderate (Spearman rank correlation coefficient 0.58), albeit significant ($p<0.001$) (figure I). Individual agreement of the two approaches based on the sub-items was fair (weighted kappa 0.35, 95% CI: 0.27-0.44) (table IV).

Table IV: Comparison of the MNA categorization obtained by the two approaches

		Nursing staff			
		Well-nourished	Risk of malnutrition	Malnutrition	Total
Resident interviews	Well-nourished	26	17	1	44
	Risk of malnutrition	25	44	4	73
	Malnutrition	0	14	7	21
	Total	51	75	12	138

Figure II: Scatter plot of the full MNA score resident vs. nursing staff

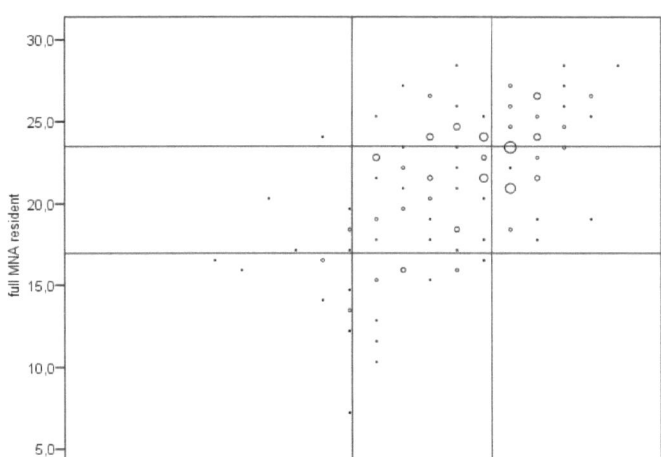

The size of bubbles indicates the frequency when scoring results of both approaches met. The lines represent the cut-off values of the three MNA categories.

Agreement between the two approaches was, apart from item H 'prescription drugs intake' (κ=0.38) and item I 'skin problems' (κ=0.21), for all additional items of the long form rated as not higher than would have been by chance distribution. Symmetry of classification distribution tests revealed, that for item K 'consumption markers for protein intake' nursing staff provided more points than residents did, while for items H 'prescription drugs intake', L 'consumption of fruits and vegetables' and item M 'fluid consumption', the residents interviews scored higher. With regard to item O addressing the estimation of the residents' nutritional status, results showed a similar distribution for the self-estimation and the estimation by the nursing staff. Here, only 2.2% (nursing staff) and 2.9% (residents) were viewed as malnourished, respectively. Nevertheless, agreement was poor (κ=0.02). With regard to the estimation of the general health status in item P, more residents than nursing staff assessed their health status as better than that of their peers (29.0% vs. 16.7%), depicting a poor agreement (κ=0.03) (table III).

Cognitive status and MNA application

A subanalysis on categorisation by the full MNA was performed for those 49 residents with a MMSE score of at least 25 points, indicating the absence of dementia. The agreement between the two approaches increased to weighted κ=0.47 (95% CI: 0.25-0.68).

MNA application and prognosis

The prognostic values of the two modes of application were evaluated with regard to mortality during a six-month follow-up period. In total 25 (12.5%) study participants deceased during this period. Table V shows the mortality rates for the different MNA categories (n=138). 19.0% of the residents categorised as malnourished by one-on-one interviews and 33.3% of those placed in this category by assessment of the nursing staff residents deceased during the follow-up. The association between mortality and the categorisation was statistically stronger for the nurses' assessment (nursing staff $p<0.001$, residents $p<0.05$; Chi^2 test).

Table V: Six-month mortality rate in the three categories of the MNA – resident interviews

	Nursing staff*	Resident*
Well-nourished	3.9%	0%
At risk of malnutrition	9.3%	12.3%
Malnutrition	33.3%	19.0%

*Significant trend of increasing mortality across the three ordinal MNA score categories (Mantel-Haenszel-Chi²: $p \leq 0.05$)

Discussion

This is the first study in nursing home residents that compared the results of the MNA applied by one-on-one interviews with the results obtained when the MNA was performed solely by the attending nursing staff. Applicability was different for these two approaches, with a lower rate for the one-on-one interviews (69.0% vs. 94.0%). The agreement of the results of the two approaches of application was tested for the MNA short form and for the full MNA. It was low for both methods, but improved when cognitively impaired participants were excluded from analysis. While mortality after six months was associated with the MNA results of both approaches, this relationship was statistically stronger for the MNA completed by the nursing staff. Notably, residents that were unable to complete the MNA in a one-to-one interview were in a markedly worse health situation, as 11 of them died during the follow-up period (44.0% of the 25 deceased participants).

The low rate of applicability of one-on-one interviews was mainly due to the high prevalence of cognitive and linguistic deficiencies that interfered with the completion of the MNA. As this screening tool was not designed with a special focus on nursing home residents but for frail elderly people in general, this problem was not specifically addressed when the MNA was developed in the early nineties (8,9). In a relevant number of subsequent studies, residents with cognitive deficits were excluded from study participation (16,29,30). Alternatively, MNA completion relied on information obtained from close relatives (29), while some authors did not even disclose how they dealt with this problem (32,37). In a study on geriatric hospital patients that did not exclude those with dementia, an applicability rate of 66.1% was reported (20), causes for non-applicability including confusion, advanced dementia, post stroke aphasia and apraxia. With regard to the long term care setting, Donini (33) reported that all MNA questions were answered completely only in 17.5% of cases. Additionally, the authors of this study could not perform the anthropometric measurements correctly in 6.2% of cases. In our study, this problem was present in only 1% of participants.

In the present study, we aimed at the inclusion of a representative sample of the nursing home population. In addition, dementia has to be regarded as one of the most relevant comorbidities with regard to malnutrition in the elderly. Therefore, we did not exclude residents with dementia from our analyses despite the above presented difficulties. The agreement between the interviews and the assessment by nursing staff was low with regard to the results of MNAsf as well as those of the full MNA. Likewise, the agreement was low for several of the MNA items that were analyzed separately. The observation that the agreement between the two approaches improved when those residents were excluded that showed dementia according to the MMSE illustrates the relevance of this frequent comorbidity for the reliability of MNA categorisation.

While it is obvious that the impairment of memory seen in dementia will generally affect the reliability of answers provided by the resident, the MNA questions that address the residents' self assessment (items O and P) may be seen as especially crucial for the application of the MNA in the nursing home setting. As their living space and their personal contacts usually become limited, many nursing home residents loose the capability to self-assess their nutritional and general health status in comparison to their peers. This observation can be applied not only to those that are affected by early stages of dementia, but also to residents with residues after cerebral ischemia and to those with Parkinson's disease. The aforementioned problems with regard to the MNA self-assessment items of institutionalized elderly persons have been addressed only by few studies yet. In a recent study by Tsai et al., the answers provided by interviews with the residents were compared to those provided by the attending nurses in a long-term care centre (11), but only in the sub-group of cognitively competent residents. Results showed that residents assessed their nutritional and health status more often as poor and that they were frequently insecure about their status than when compared to the nursing staff's assessment. In another study substitution of the two questions addressing self-assessment was suggested and tested (33).

In the MNA user guide (38) it is recommended to ask the patient's caregiver or the attending nursing staff member, if the resident himself is not capable to provide an adequate answer to MNA questions. But it is not an easy task to decide when to shift the MNA application from the interview type to the exclusive assessment by the attending nurse or caregiver. In most cases, the resident's capability to complete the MNA in a reliable way will decrease gradually and so it will not be possible to provide a clear threshold when the mode of application should be changed. Therefore, we suggest that in nursing homes with a high prevalence of dementia, the MNA should routinely be completed by the attending nurses.

The inter-rater reliability of this mode of MNA application has been tested in two studies (31,35). It was proven moderate, respectively good with kappa values of 0.53 and 0.78. The results for several MNA sub-items were more diverse.

In the original publication on the MNA, all participants classified as "normal" were still alive after one year of follow-up, while 24% of the patients "at risk" and 48% of the "malnourished" died during this period (36). When assessing the ability of the full MNA to predict in-hospital and long-term mortality in old hospitalised patients, Kagansky and co-workers found a significant correlation between the full MNA and survival rates after 2.7 years (30). Mortality in malnourished participants was 3-fold higher than in well-nourished ones (38.7% vs. 12.5%). Persson et al. (34) reported a 50% mortality rate in malnourished elderly after one year. In the study by Tsai et al. (11), it was shown that the MNA by caregiver's assessment predicted six-month follow-up mortality in cognitively impaired elderly. The results of our study add to the scarce longitudinal data currently available for MNA application in the nursing home setting. In the present study, association with mortality was highest in those categorised as malnourished which could be shown for both approaches (table 5). Nevertheless, this relationship was statistically more profound for the assessment by the nursing staff with a higher positive predictive value. As malnutrition is closely related to mortality among the elderly, this observation enforces that the assessment by nursing staff is superior.

The lack of applicability of the MNA in residents with percutaneous endoscopic gastrostomies (PEG) should not be interpreted as a fault of this screening instrument as these residents are commonly regarded as being at risk of malnutrition in any case. As a consequence, they are supposed to have a nutritional plan with fixed intakes and to be subjected to regular monitoring of their nutritional status.

Conclusion

The applicability of the MNA in nursing homes with a high percentage of cognitively impaired residents has to be considered as limited if performed by one-on-one interviews. As the risk of malnutrition is high in this sub-group and nutritional screening in this population has therefore to be regarded as mandatory, we suggest that the MNA should be performed routinely by the nursing staff. In this regard, it has to be considered that a valid MNA can only be provided by the nursing staff when there is thorough knowledge of the different aspects of the resident's life. With regard to the use of the MNA in scientific research, it has to be stressed that authors should regularly provide information on the method used for MNA application. This will be necessary to ensure the comparability of epidemiological and interventional data in the nursing home setting.

References II

1 CEDERHOLM T, JAGREN C, HELLSTROM K: Outcome of protein-energy malnutrition in elderly medical patients. Am J Med 1995;98:67-74.
2 DEY DK, ROTHENBERG E, SUNDH V, BOSAEUS I, STEEN B: Body Mass Index, weight change and mortality in the elderly. A 15 year longitudinal population study of 70 y olds. Eur J Clin Nutr 2001;55:482-92.
3 AMARANTOS E, MARTINEZ A, DWYER J: Nutrition and Quality of Life in older Adults. J Gerontol 2001;56A:54-64.
4 KONDRUP J, ALLISON SP, ELIA M, VELLAS B, PLAUTH M.: ESPEN Guidelines for Nutrition Screening 2002. Clin Nutr 2002;22(4):415-421.
5 PAULY L, STEHLE P, VOLKERT D: Nutritional Situation of elderly nursing home residents. Z Gerontol Geriat 2007;40: 3-12.
6 BAUER JM, KAISER M, ANTHONY P, GUIGOZ Y, SIEBER CC: The Mini Nutritional Assessment-Its History, Today's Practice, and Future Perspectives. Nutr Clin Pract 2008;23(4):388-96.
7 MORLEY JE AND THOMAS DR: Anorexia and aging: pathophysiology. Nutrition 1999;15:499-503.
8 GUIGOZ Y, VELLAS B, GARRY PJ: Assessing the Nutritional Status of the elderly. The Mini Nutritional Assessment as Part of the Geriatric Evaluation. Nutrition reviews 1996;54:59-65.
9 GUIGOZ Y, VELLAS B, GARRY PJ: Mini Nutritional Assessment: a practical assessment tool for grading the nutritional state of elderly patients. Facts Res Gerontol 1994;(2):15-60.
10 VELLAS B, GARRY PJ, GUIGOZ Y: Mini Nutritional Assessment (MNA): Research and Practice in the Elderly. Nestle nutrition Workshop Series Clinical & Performance Programme, Nestec Ltd; Vervey/S. Karger AG, Basel ©,1999;1:3-12.
11 TSAI A AND KU PY: Population-specific Mini Nutritional Assessment effectively predicts the nutritional state and follow-up mortality of institutionalized elderly Taiwanese regardless of cognitive status. Br Nutr 2007;1-7.
12 WIBKY K, EK AC, CRISTENSSON L: The two-step Mini Nutritional Assessment procedure in community resident homes. J Clin Nurs 2008,1211-1218.

13 ESSED NH, VAN STAVEREN WA, KOK FJ, DE GRAAF C: No effect of 16 weeks flavor enhancement on dietary intake and nutritional status of nursing home elderly. Appetite 2007;48(1):29-36.

14 SOUMINEN MH, SANDELIN E, SOINI H, PITKALA KH: How well do nurses recognize malnutrition in elderly patients? Eur J Clin Nutr. Epub 2007;Sep 19.

15 DION N, COTART JL, RABILLOUD M: Correction of nutrition test errors for more accurate quantification of the link between dental health and malnutrition. Nutrition 2007;23(4):301-307.

16 NORMAN K, SMOLINER C, VALENTINI L, LOCHS H, PIRLICH M: Is bioelectrical impedance vector analysis of value in the elderly with malnutrition and impaired functionality? Nutrition 2007;23(7-8):564-569.

17 NIJS KA, DE GRAAF C, SIEBELINK E ET AL.: Effect of family-style meals on energy intake and risk of malnutrition Dutch nursing home residents: a randomized controlled trial. J Gerontol A Biol Sci Med Sci 2006;61(9):935-942.

18 SOINI H, MUURINEN S, ROUTASALO P, ET AL.: Oral and nutritional status-is the MNA a useful tool for dental clinics? J Nutr Health Aging 2006;10(6):495-499; discussion 500-501.

19 WOJSZEL ZB.: Determinants of nutritional status of older people in long-term care settings on the sample of nursing homes in Bialystok. Adv Med Sci 2006;51:168-173.

20 BAUER JM, VOGL T, WICKLEIN S, TRÖGNER J, MÜHLBERG W, SIEBER CC: Comparison of the Mini Nutritional Assessment, Subjective Global Assessment, and Nutritional Risk Screening (NRS 2002) for nutritional screening and assessment in geriatric hospital patients. Z Gerontol Geriatr. 2005;38:322-327.

21 FOLSTEIN MF, FOLSTEIN S, MCHUGH PR: Mini Mental State: a practical method for grading cognitive state of patients for he clinician. J Psychiatr Res 1975;12:189-198

22 LESHER EL AND BERRYHILL JS: Validation of the Geriatric Depression Scale-short form amoung inpatients. J Clin Psychol1994;50:256-60.

23 ARBEITSGEMEINSCHAFT FÜR KLINISCHE ERNÄHRUNG (AKE). www.ake-nutrition.at: 22.07.2008

24 CHUMLEA W, ROCHE A, STEINBAUGH M: estimating stature from knee height for persons 60-90 years of age. J Am Geriatr Soc 1985;33:116-120.

25 CHUMLEA WW, GUO S, WHOLIHAN K, COCKRAM D, KUCZMARSKI RJ, JOHNSON CL: Stature predictions equations for elderly non-Hispanic white, non-Hispanic black and Mexican American persons developed from NHANES-III data. J Amer dietet Assoc 1998;98:137-142.
26 MAHONEY FI AND BARTHEL DW: Functional Evaluation: The Barthel Index. Maryland State Medical Journal 1965;14: 61-65.
27 RUBENSTEIN LZ, HARKER JO, SALVA A, GUIGOZ Y, VELLAS B: Screening for undernutrition in geriatric practice: developing the short-form Mini-Nutritional Assessment (MNA-SF). J Gerontol A Biol Sci Med Sci 2001;56:M366-M372.
28 COHEN A: Coefficient of agreement for nominal scales. Educ Psychol Meas 1960;19:3-11.
29 HENGSTERMANN S, NIECZAJ R, STEINHAGEN-THIESSEN E, SCHULZ R-J: Which are the most efficient items of the Mini Nutritional Assessment in multimorbid patients? J Nutr Health Aging 2008;12(2):117-122.
30 KAGANSKY N, BERNER Y, KOREN-MORAG N, PERELMAN L, KNOBLER H, LEVY S: Poor nutritional habits are predictors of poor outcome in very old hospitalized patients. Am J Clin Nutr 2005;82:784-91.
31 BLEDA MJ, BOLIBAR I, PARÉS R, SALVÁ A: Reliability of the Mini Nutritional Assessment (MNA) in institutionalized elderly people, J Nutr Health Aging 2002;6(2):134-137.
32 ÖDLUND OLIN A, KOOCHEK A, LJUNGQVIST O, CEDERHOLM T: Nutritional status, well-being and functional ability in frail elderly service flat residents. Eur J Clin Nutr 2005;59:263-270.
33 DONINI LM, DE FELICE MR, TASSI L, DE BERNADINI L, PINTO A, GIUSTINI AM, CANNELLA C: A "Proportional and objective score" for the Mini Nutritional Assessment in a long term geriatric care. J Nutr Health Aging 2002;6(2):141-146.
34 PERSSON MD, BRISMAR KE, KATZARSKI KS, NORDENSTRÖM J, CEDERHOLM TE: Nutritional status using mini nutritional assessment and subjective global assessment predict mortality in geriatric patients. J Am Geriatr Soc 2002;50;1996-2002.
35 NEUMANN SA, MILLER MD, DANIELS LA, AHERN M, CROTTY M: Mini Nutritional Assessment in geriatric rehabilitation: Inter-rater reliability and relationship to body composition and nutritional biochemistry 2007;64:179-185.

36 GUIGOZ Y AND VELLAS B: Test d'evaluation de l'etat nutritionnel de la personne agée: le Mini Nutirtionel Assessment (MNA). Med Hyg. 1995;53:1965-1969.
37 KULNIK D, ELMADFA I: Assessment of the Nutritional Situation of elderly Nursing home Residents in Vienna. Ann Nutr Metab 2008;52:51-53.
38 NESTLÉ, www.mna.elderly.com;10/2008.

Chapter three

Specific blood markers of nutritional status in nursing home residents

Introduction

In the course of aging, the capacity and selectivity of physiological functions is continuously decreasing. The extent of this loss of function is different from individual to individual; generally, the human body has sufficient reserves to maintain a normal metabolism over a long period of time. It is known that body composition is changing (loss of muscle mass, increase of fat mass) with increasing age (MORLEY 1997). In combination with a decreased physical activity, this leads to lower energy expenditure. Consequently, the recommendations for energy intake in the elderly are less than for middle-aged adults. The metabolic needs for micronutrients, however, are similar to adults or are even higher because of age-associated metabolic changes or chronic diseases (DACH 2000). It is, thus, mandatory that elderly preferably consume food with low energy but high nutrient density. Unfortunately, this guideline is hardly followed in the general older population. Moreover, comorbidities may further contribute to impaired absorption, transport, metabolism, and excretion of nutrients (DREWNOWSKI AND SCHULTZ 2001).

Altogether, this leads to an increased risk of malnutrition in frail and dependent elderly people. It is known that an inadequate endogenous availability of micronutrients reduces quality of life and functionality, and contributes to enhanced morbidity and mortality rates (BROWNIE 2006). To detect special needs of population groups, as for example the elderly, the assessment of the micronutrient status is mandatory and provides a basis for recommendations in regard to early recognition and counteraction of deficiencies.

Different methods are available to determine individual micronutrient status. The measurement of blood parameters is an invasive and expensive, but also exact method to analyze the nutritional status of a person in general or with regard to a specific nutrient or vitamin. In several studies, a low serum status or a low intake of micronutrients of the community-dwelling elderly was associated with a decrease in different parameters, such as functionality, cognition and an increase of morbidity and mortality (BARTALI ET AL. 2008, BARTALI ET AL. 2006, BLE ET AL. 2006, BUIJSSE ET AL. 2005, CESARI ET AL. 2004, FLETCHER ET AL. 2003, HOUSTON ET AL. 2007, MORRIS ET AL. 2002, SEMBA ET AL. 2006). Longitudinal data on nursing home residents regarding the monitoring of nutrient blood level are scarce. Moreover, the associations between nutritional blood status, functional parameters, and mortality are not known in this group of elderly.

This study, thus, aims at describing the nutrient blood status of α-tocopherol, retinol, vitamin D, ß-carotene, folate, vitamin B_{12} and albumin in elderly nursing home residents at the beginning of the study (t_0) and after one year of observation (t_{12}, with regard to α-tocopherol, retinol, vitamin D, ß-carotene), also focusing the prevalence of nutrient deficiencies. The nutrient status of tube-fed residents and normally fed residents was compared. Furthermore, the study aims at analyzing associations between nutrient blood levels, functionality and mortality in this population.

Methods

Subjects

All residents (age $\geq$ 65 y.) of two municipal nursing homes in Nuremberg, Germany, were approached to participate in the present study between June 2007 and December 2008. Residents with end-stages diseases were excluded. Informed consent was obtained from all participating residents or their legal proxies. The study protocol was approved by the ethics committees of the Friedrich-Alexander-University of Erlangen-Nuremberg, Germany, and the Rheinische Friedrich-Wilhelms-University of Bonn, Germany.

Baseline characteristics

All general data, including information about gender, age, care level, smoking habits and PEG feeding, were collected from the nursing staff or the residents' files. According to the German system (2007) the level of care is either level 0 (no need of care yet), 1 (low), 2 (high) or 3 (highest care needs). A physician recorded type and number of medications from the medical files. The cognitive status of each participant was evaluated using the Mini Mental State Examination (MMSE) (FOLSTEIN ET AL. 1975). The emotional status was tested by the short form of the Geriatric Depression Scale (15 questions) (SHEIK AND YESAVAGE 1986), validated by Lesher and Berryhill in 1994 (LESHER AND BERRYHILL 1994).

Nutrition related clinical symptoms

Information on wound healing disorder, decubitus ulcer, exsiccosis, oedema, nausea, vomiting, constipation, diarrhoea and the presence and degree of anorexia, swallowing and chewing difficulties were recorded as assessed by nursing staff.

Morbidity

A physician of the study team recorded all chronic and acute diseases as well as type and number of medications from the medical files.

General nutritional status - MNA and anthropometry

The nutritional status was determined by the Mini Nutritional Assessment® (MNA, MINI NUTRITIONAL ASSESSMENT 2009), a screening tool specifically developed for the identification of malnutrition or its risk the elderly (GUIGOZ ET AL. 1994, GUIGOZ ET AL. 1996, BAUER ET AL. 2008). Except for its anthropometric items, the MNA was performed by the nursing staff, due to the high prevalence of cognitive impairment of the participants.

Anthropometric assessment performed by a nutrition scientist included body mass index (BMI), mid-arm circumference, calf circumference and triceps skinfold thickness. BMI was calculated by weight (kg) (to the nearest 0.1 kg with a weigh chair type Arjo CFA 2000) divided by body height squared (m^2). Height measurement was carried out by measuring knee height, using a knee height caliper from the Austrian Society of Clinical Nutrition (AKE), according to the method described elsewhere (CHUMLEA ET AL. 1985). The corresponding body height was calculated using the formula of Chumlea et al. (CHUMLEA ET AL. 1998). Measurements of mid-arm circumference and calf circumference were carried out with a flexible measuring tape and were recorded to the nearest 0.1 cm. Mid-arm circumference was measured on the left side at the mid-point between the tip of the shoulder and the tip of the elbow between olecranon process and acromion. Triceps skinfold thickness was determined at the same position with a GPM skinfold caliper to the nearest 0.2 mm (DKSH Switzerland Ltd.). Calf circumference was measured in a supine or sitting position on the left side at the widest point without compressing the subcutaneous tissue. The mean value from two consecutive measurements was recorded for all parameters. Participants with enteral nutrition were noted by the study team.

Functional parameters

Measurement of handgrip strength (HGS) was carried out using a vigorimeter (by Martin, Tuttlingen, Germany), recording to the nearest 0.2 kPa. For the timed 'up and go' test (TUG), the residents were asked to stand up from an armchair, to walk three meters, turn around, return to the chair, and sit down again. The time needed was measured to the nearest full second. The Index of activities of daily living (ADL) according to Barthel (MAHONY AND BARTHEL 1965) was recorded by the nursing staff. Residents with a score between 65 and 100 points were considered as independent, residents with a score between 35 and 60 points in need of assistance and residents scoring < 35 points were considered to require a high level of care.

Specific markers of nutritional status - Blood analyses

Fasten blood samples were taken in EDTA tubes in the morning between 6:30 and 8:00 a.m. Within one hour, the blood was centrifuged, the plasma obtained aliquoted and stored at -80°.

Serum folate, B_{12}, cholesterol and *albumin* were processed similar to EDTA tubes and analyzed at the Institute of Clinical Chemistry and Laboratory Medicine of the Clinic Nuremberg. Measurement of folate was performed on the Cobas e 601 immunoanalyzer with the folate III assay (Roche Diagnostics Mannheim, Germany). Vitamin B_{12} was measured on the Cobas e 601 immunoanalyzer with the vitamin B_{12} assay (Roche Diagnostics, Mannheim, Germany). Both methods are based on an electrochemiluminescence immunoassay method (ECLIA). Cholesterol was measured with the Cholesterol-oxidase method on an Olympus Clinical Chemistry analyzer AU 2700 (Olympus, Hamburg, Germany).

Albumin was measured nephelometrically on an Image Nephelometer (Beckman Coulter, Krefeld, Germany).

25(OH)D was analyzed by ELISA (Immuno Diagnostic Systems Ltd, Germany). *α-tocopherol, ß-carotene* and *retinol* in plasma were analyzed by HPLC according to VUILLEUMIER ET AL.1983. Briefly, 400 µl of plasma were mixed with the same amount of ethanol to precipitate protein. Subsequently, vitamins were extracted with 200 µl n-hexane. The hexane phase was analyzed at 292 nm (α-tocopherol, retinol) and at 450 nm (ß-carotene) after separation on a nucleosil 100-5 CN, 250x4.0 mm column (Macherey and Nagel, Dueren). For quantification, apo-ß-carotenal was used as an internal standard. Cut-off values to define a low blood level were applied as follows:

Vitamin D	< 10 nmol/l: severe vitamin D deficiency, 10-< 25 nmol/l: moderate deficiency, 25-< 50 nmol/l: light deficiency, 50-< 75 nmol/l: still suboptimal, 75 nmol/l: optimal status (LIPS ET AL. 2006, BISCHOFF-FERRARI ET AL. 2006, ZITTERMANN 2006, BASHA ET AL. 2000, PEACOCK 1993)
Albumin	> 60 years < 3.4 mg/dl; > 70 years < 3.3 mg/dl > 80 years < 3.1 mg/dl; > 90 years < 3.0 mg/dl (JOHNSON ET AL. 1996)
Retinol	$\leq$ 1.34 µmol/l men, $\leq$ 1.02 µmol/l women (HESEKER ET AL. 1992)
ß-carotene	$\leq$ 0.18 µmol/l (HESEKER ET AL. 1992)
Vitamin B_{12}	< 141 pmol/l (kit manufacturer, Roche Diagnostics, Mannheim, Germany)
Folate	< 7.5 nmol/l (WRIGHT ET AL 1998)
α- tocopherol	$\leq$ 17.7 µmol/l (HESEKER ET AL. 1992)
α- tocopherol/ cholesterol ratio	< 2.2 µmol/mmol (MORRISSEY ET AL. 1993)

Follow-up examination

All questionnaires, geriatric assessments, measurements of anthropometry and functionality and the analysis of blood samples, except for vitamin B_{12}, folate, cholesterol and albumin, were repeated after twelve months (t_{12}). Data on supplementation of vitamin D during the study period and data on mortality within one year of observation were collected from the residents' medical records.

Statistics

Statistical analysis was performed using SPSS© version 17.0 (SPSS for Windows, SPSS Inc., Chicago, IL, USA) Results are given in mean ± standard deviation (SD) in normally distributed data, as median and range (5th-95th percentile) and in box plots in non-normal distributed data. T-tests for independent and dependent samples, respectively, were used to compare differences in variables between baseline and follow-up or between different groups, in case of normally distributed data. Non-normal distributed variables of dependent variables (t_0 and t_{12}) were compared using the Wilcoxon-signed-rank test. Non-normal distributed variables of two independent variables (deceased and survivors) were compared using the Mann-Whitney-U test.

Non-normal distributed variables of n independent variables were compared using the Kruskall-Wallis test. The Chi^2 test was used to test whether or not an observed frequency distribution differs from a theoretical distribution. The correlations among continuous variables were assessed using the Spearman-Rho correlation coefficient. Statistical tests were performed two-sided. Chi^2 trend test was used to test the ordinal scale of mortality in the vitamin D categories. A p-value ≤ 0.05 was regarded as significant.

Results

Baseline characteristics

Table VI presents summarized baseline characteristics (gender, age, MMSE, GDS and MNA score, anthropometric and functional measurements) of the 200 participants (participation rate: 62%). General data of all participants in t_0 regarding the level of care, number of regular taken drugs including supplements, smoking habits, and the prevalence of tube-feeding (PEG), as well as nutritional status-dependent symptoms (e.g. wound healing disorder) and symptoms which influence the nutritional status (e.g. nausea, vomiting, etc) are presented in table VII.

Table VI: Baseline characteristics of all participants I

Parameter		n
Gender		
women		147
men		53
Age [y]	85.5 (±7.8)°	200
MMSE [points/ max. 30]	19 (0-29)⁺	183
GDS [points/ max. 15]	4.5 (0.2-12.0)⁺	142
MNA [points/ max. 30]	21.5 (13.7-27.0)⁺	188
BMI [kg/m²]	26.3 (±5.3)°	200
MAC [cm]	28.5 (±4.5)°	200
CC [cm]	32.7 (±5.0)°	197
Handgrip strength [kPa]		
women	36.8 (±19.3)°	116
men	41.9 (±16.7)°	48
Timed 'up & go' [sec]	26 (12-61.9)⁺	85
ADL [points/100]	45 [0-90]⁺	200

⁺median (5th-95th percentile), °mean (±SD)

Table VII: Baseline characteristics of all participants II

	n	%
Care level		
0	8	4.0
1	75	37.5
2	85	42.5
3	32	16.0
Number of drugs/day		
0	3	1.5
1-3	52	26.0
4-6	84	42.0
7-10	52	26.0
>10	9	4.5
Cigarette smoking habits		
non-smoker	194	97.0
current smoker	6	3.0
PEG	11	5.5
Symptoms relating/influencing nutritional status		
Wound healing disorder	11	5.5
Decubitus ulcers		
degree 1	4	2.0
degree 2	1	0.5
degree 3	6	3.0
degree 4	3	1.5
no	186	93.0
Exsiccosis	9	4.5
Oedema	56	28.0
Nausea	24	12.0
Vomiting	15	7.5
Constipation	64	32.0
Diarrhea	17	8.5
Anorexia		
severe	7	3.5
medium	14	7.0
light	45	22.5
no	127	63.5
missing	7	3.5
Chewing difficulties		
severe	7	3.5
medium	6	3.0
light	13	6.5
no	168	84.0
missing	6	3.0
Swallowing difficulties		
severe	11	5.5
medium	4	2.0
light	8	4.0
no	173	86.5
missing	4	2.0

Morbidity

Out of 200 nursing home residents, 76.5% suffered from hypertension, 74.0% from heart failure and 36% from diabetes mellitus. Figure III shows the prevalence of the most frequent chronic diseases in nursing home residents. In median, participants suffered from four diseases concomitantly.

Follow-up

Forty-seven residents deceased within one year, 14 dropped out. In several residents only incomplete assessments were possible. Baseline characteristics and follow-up data of the survivors are opposed in table VIII. MMSE score, MAC, CC and HGS (only women) showed a significant decline within twelve months.

Table VIII: Baseline and follow-up characteristics of survivors

Parameter	t_o	t_{12}	n	p
Gender women			115	
men			38	
Age [y]	85.2 (±8.3)		153	
MMSE [points/ max. 30]	20 (0-29)⁺	19 (0-30)⁺	123	§0.001
GDS [points/max. 15]	4.0 (0-12.0)⁺	4.0 (1-11.3)⁺	93	§0.640
MNA [points/max. 30]	22 (14.0-27.3)⁺	21.5 (11.7-27.0)⁺	127	§0.363
BMI [kg/m²]	26.8 (±5.4)°	26.6 (±5.8)°	139	#0.281
MAC [cm]	28.9 (±4.5)°	27.5 (±4.4)°	135	#0.000
CC [cm]	33.2 (±5.1)°	32.8 (±5.4)°	132	#0.020
Handgrip strength [kPa]				
women	38.5 (±19.1)°	34.8 (±20.9)°	79	#0.004
men	41.8 (±17.1)°	40.7 (±19.4)°	31	#0.264
Timed 'up & go' [sec]	24 (10.7-46.5)⁺	26 (10.5-53.0)⁺	49	§0.360
ADL [points/100]	45 (0-90)⁺	40 (0-90)⁺	139	§0.280

⁺median (5th-95th percentile), °mean (± SD), §Wilcoxon-signed-rank or #t-test

Figure III: Prevalence of relevant chronic diseases in nursing home residents (t_0)

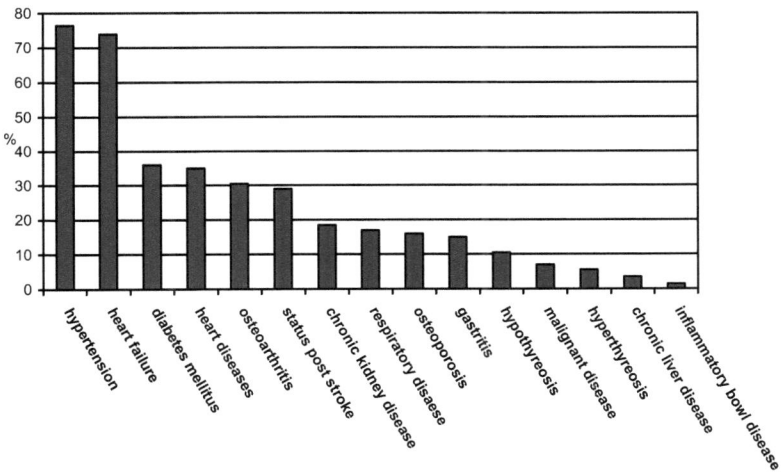

Specific markers of nutritional status

Blood was taken from 186 residents at t_0. The highest rate of deficiency (< 25 nmol/l) was calculated for vitamin D (68.3%); only 0.5% of the participants had an inadequate α-tocopherol/cholesterol ratio (table IX and figure IV). Figure V presents the number of deficiencies per resident. The majority showed a deficiency of one of the observed blood markers. No resident showed low levels in all seven analyzed parameters, 15.7% of the residents had no deficiency.

Table IX: Cut-off values and prevalence of low nutrient levels respectively nutrient deficiencies at t_0

	Cut-offs	Prevalence %
25(OH)D [nmol/l]	< 25.0	68.3
Retinol [µmol/l] men	≤ 1.34	47.1
Albumin [g/dl]	Age-adapted	26.0
Retinol [µmol/l] women	≤ 1.02	17.0
ß-Carotene [µmol/l]	≤ 0.18	9.7
B_{12} [pmol/l]	< 141	8.6
Folate [nmol/l]	< 7.5	6.5
α-Tocopherol [µmol/l	≤ 17.7	5.9
<u>α-Tocopherol [µmol]</u> Cholesterol [mmol]	< 2.2	0.5

Figure IV: Number of nutrient deficiencies at t_0

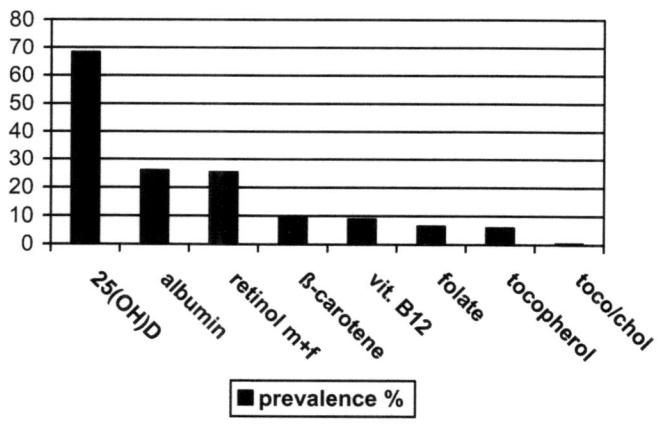

m male, f female

Figure V: Number of nutrient deficiencies per resident (t_0)

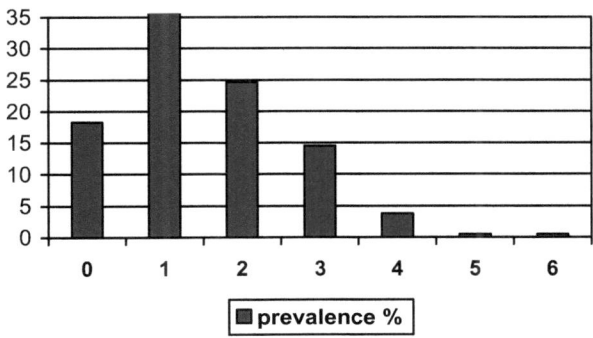

Follow-up data

In 120 residents, blood samples could be taken after one year. A second analysis was accomplished for retinol, ß-carotene, vitamin D and α-tocopherol. Due to financial reasons no second blood analysis was done for albumin, vitamin B_{12}, folate and cholesterol.

Retinol levels decreased significantly within one year, as well as the vitamin D level of residents not receiving vitamin D supplementation. Contrary, the vitamin D level of residents who supplemented this vitamin (22%) increased significantly (table X). Blood levels of vitamin D, retinol, ß-carotene and α-tocopherol at t_0 and t_{12} of residents with blood sampling at both points of time are presented in figure VI.

Table X: Blood parameters in t_0 and t_{12}

Nutrient	t_0°	n	t_{12}°	n	p[$]
Retinol [µmol/l]	1.53 (0.7-2.7)	186	1.38 (0.6-2.5)	121	0.029
25(OH)D [nmol/l] all	20.8 (12.4-67.5)	186	21.8 (10.3-106.7)	121	0.102
no supplementation	20.7 (12.5-55.5)	145	17.8 (9.5-59.5)	88	0.000
supplementation (t_0-t_{12})	20.8 (11.7-144.6)	41	79.6 (28.2-128.5)	33	0.000
ß-Carotene [µmol/l]	0.55 (0.13-1.29)	186	0.6 (0.1-2.1)	120	0.648
α-Tocopherol [µmol/l]	29.1 (16.5-52)	186	30.9 (16.3-47.1)	121	0.927
Folate [nmol/l]	14.2 (6.8-44.3)	185	not available	-	-
B$_{12}$ [pmol/l]	267.8 (125.8-424.8)	185	not available	-	-
Cholesterol [mmol/l]	5.3 (3.5-7.3)	185	not available	-	-
α-Tocopherol [µmol] Cholesterol [mmol]	5.5 (3.6-8.9)	185	not available	-	-
Albumin [g/dl]	3.4 (2.7-4.1)	185	not available	-	-

°data are given in median (5th-95th percentile), [$]Wilcoxon-signed-rank test, comparison of the residents' data available for both times

Figure VI: Box plots of nutrient levels of survivors at t_0 and t_{12} (n=121, ß-carotene n=120)

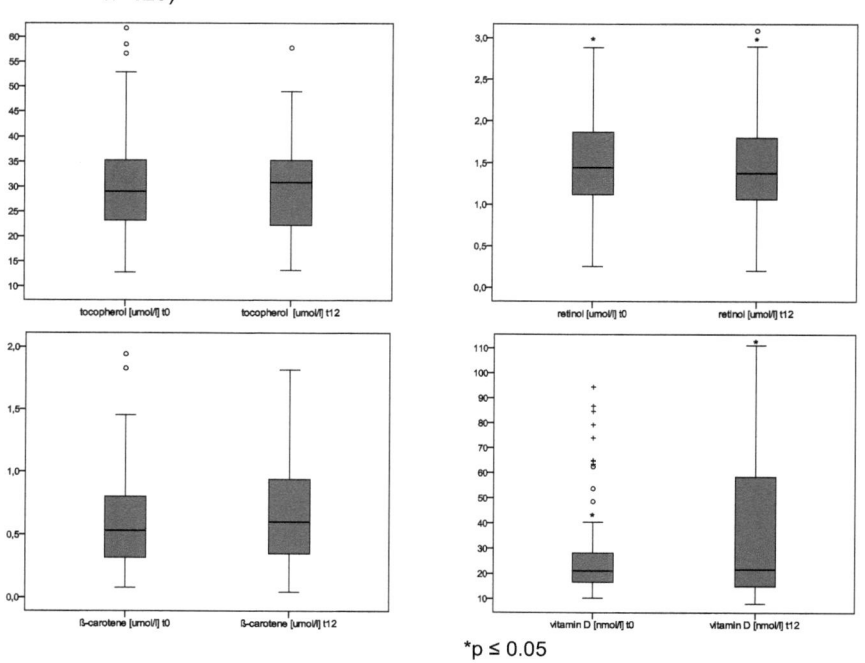

*p ≤ 0.05

Enteral nutrition

11 residents were fed by PEG. Table XI shows the analysis of the nutrient blood level of tube-fed residents in comparison to non-tube-fed residents. The α-tocopherol/cholesterol quotient showed a significantly higher value in the tube-fed population. Cholesterol was significantly lower. Furthermore, 25(OH)D and the folate level were significantly higher in residents with PEG. Four of the tube-fed residents deceased during the study. There were no significant differences of mortality between tube-fed and oral-fed residents (Chi^2-test, p=0.357).

Table XI: Comparison of blood level (non tube-fed vs. tube-fed)

Nutrient	Non-tube-fed°	n	tube-fed°	n	p$^\$$
Cholesterol [mmol/l]	5.4 (3.5-7.7)	174	4.7 (2.6-5.8)	11	0.011
α-tocopherol [µmol] Cholesterol [mmol]	5.4 (3.6-8.5)	174	6.9 (5.9-9.6)	11	0.000
25(OH)D [nmol/l]	20.3 (12.3-63.9)	174	53.8 (27.4-73.0)	11	0.000
Folate [nmol/l]	14.0 (6.7-37.2)	174	33.6 (22.2-48.3)	11	0.000
α-tocopherol [µmol/l]	28.8 (16.1-53.8)	174	32.1 (18.6-41.9)	11	0.247
Retinol [µmol/l]	1.42 (0.7-2.7)	174	1.6 (0.7-2.8)	11	0.763
ß-carotene [µmol/l]	0.55 (0.13-1.28)	174	0.71 (0.07-3.7)	11	0.568
B$_{12}$ [pmol/l]	266.0 (124.3-586.2)	174	298.1 (139.4-618.1)	11	0.146
Albumin [g/dl]	3.4 (2.7-4.1)	174	3.2 (2.7-4.1)	11	0.295

°data are given in median (5th-95th percentile), $^\$$Mann-Whitney-U test (exact)

Comparison of survivors and non-survivors

Table XII presents the blood levels at t_0 of the surviving and deceased residents. A higher level of nutrient status in the group of survivors, except for ß-carotene and vitamin B$_{12}$ levels was observed but without reaching statistical significance. Figure VII shows the prevalence of low levels, stratified for surviving and deceased residents at t_0. No significant difference was observed (Chi^2-test, p>0.05).

Table XII: Nutrient status of deceased and survivors at t_0

Nutrient	Survivors°	n	Deceased°	n	p$^\$$
α-Tocopherol [µmol/l]	29.3 (16.9-52.9)	139	28.0 (15.6-53.2)	46	0.470
α-Tocopherol [µmol] Cholesterol [mmol]	5.5 (3.6-9.6)	139	5.5 (3.9-8.6)	46	0.943
Cholesterol [mmol/l]	5.4 (3.5-7.7)	139	5.1 (3.2-7.1)	46	0.584
Retinol [µmol/ml]	1.5 (0.7-2.8)	139	1.4 (0.7-3.5)	46	0.201
ß-Carotene [µmol/l]	0.5 (0.1-1.3)	139	0.6 (0.1-1.2)	46	0.602
25(OH)D [nmol/l]	21.3 (12.4-75.2)	139	18.4 (11.6-53.1)	46	0.131
Folate [nmol/l]	14.2 (7.0-45.9)	139	14.0 (6.6-38.0)	46	0.348
Vitamin B_{12} [pmol/l]	266.3 (123.2-645.6)	139	290.3 (140.0-578.7)	46	0.134
Albumin [g/dl]	3.4 (2.7-4.1)	139	3.3 (2.7-4.1)	46	0.273

°median (5th-95th percentile), $^\$$Mann-Whitney-U test (exact)

Figure VII: Prevalence of low blood levels (survivors vs. deceased) at t_0

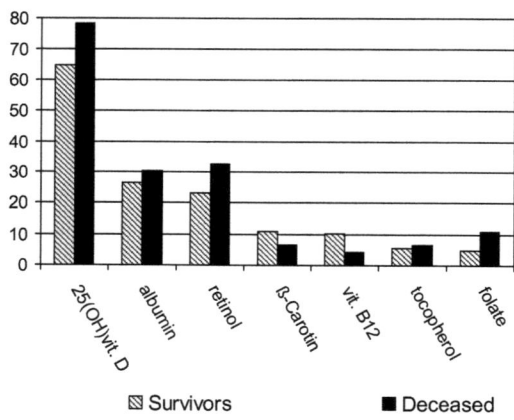

Vitamin D and survival

68.3% of the residents showed 25(OH)D level between 10 - < 25 nmol/l, 22.6% showed higher levels between 25 - < 50 nmol/l. Levels between 50 - < 75 nmol/l or ≥ 75 nmol/l were determined for 5.4% and 3.8% respectively. No resident suffered from severe vitamin D deficiency (< 10 nmol/l). The cumulative survival of these groups is presented in figure VIII.

Figure VIII: Survival (cum.) in the vitamin D groups (t_0)

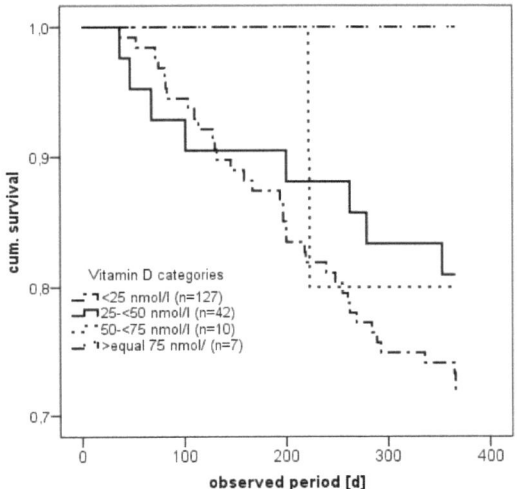

Functionality and blood level

25(OH)D level was significantly associated with handgrip strength (Spearman's Rho 0.219; p=0.007) and Barthel-ADL score (0.197; p=0.007). Similarly, a significant correlation has been observed between retinol status and Barthel-ADL score (0.161; p≤0.05) as well as folate and the time needed in the timed 'up and go' test (-0.299; p≤0.05). Additionally, handgrip strength and ADL were significantly correlated with albumin status (0.263; p≤0.001 and 0.351; p≤0.001).

Discussion

To my knowledge, this is the first longitudinal study without interventional approach, analyzing specific nutritional blood markers of nursing home residents and relating these data with parameters of functionality and mortality.

Current cross-sectional studies generally confirm an adequate supply of most micronutrients (vitamins and minerals) in elderly people living in the community (BLE ET AL. 2006, SEMBA ET AL. 2006, VOLKERT AND STEHLE 1999). Insufficient serum levels have only been observed for vitamin D, B_{12} and folate (SEMBA ET AL. 2006, BJOERKEGREN AND SVAERDSUDD 2001, BAIK AND RUSSELL 1999, BISCHOFF ET AL. 1999, KARG AND GEDRICH 1996). Data on the micronutrient status of elderly nursing home residents are available (GONZALEZ-GROSS ET AL. 2007, MONGET ET AL. 1996, SAHYOUN ET AL. 1988, HARRILL AND CERVONE 1977), but scarce. So far, most attention has been given to community-dwelling elderly or to an interventional approach (MOREIRA-PFRIMER ET AL. 2009, BARTALI ET AL. 2008, BROE ET AL. 2007, BLE ET AL. 2006, SEMBA ET AL. 2006, BUIJSSE ET AL. 2005, BISCHOFF-FERRARI ET AL. 2004). Generally, institutionalized elderly showed lower blood levels of nutrients in comparison to independent living elderly (LOEWIK ET AL 1992).

Description of blood levels

In the context of the following description of nutritional blood markers it has to be taken into account, that the present study is limited by missing data about nutritional intake. Consequently, no statement can be given regarding the influence of nutrient intake on blood level.

In the present study, the highest prevalence of blood level deficiency was shown for vitamin D. An increased prevalence of vitamin D deficiency with increasing dependency was already shown before (PAPAPETROU ET AL. 2008). The mean vitamin D level was lower than in several previous nursing home studies (BROE ET AL. 2007, WOUTERS-WESSELING ET AL. 2002, ALLSUP ET AL. 2004, PEREZ-LLAMAS ET AL. 2008). Community-dwelling, independent living elderly show higher levels of vitamin D (HOUSTON ET AL. 2007, BISCHOFF ET AL. 1999, BISCHOFF-FERRARI ET AL. 2004, BARTALI ET AL. 2006, HESEKER ET AL. 1992) and lower prevalence of vitamin D deficiencies, respectively (VISSER ET AL. 2006), which might be explained by the higher physical performance of these elderly and the resulting greater ability to go outside. In the present study, supplementation of vitamin D, resulted in significantly increased 25(OH)D levels. This positive effect of supplementation has already been shown in several nursing home studies (KUWABARA ET AL. 2009, HIMENAO ET AL. 2009, LIPS ET AL. 1988) and the community as well (LIPS ET AL. 1988, HARRIS AND DAWSON-HUGHES 2002).

Vitamin D is involved in the pathogenesis of osteoporosis and additionally influences muscle function. The present results (*'functionality and blood level'*) confirm the association of higher vitamin D levels with functionality, displayed by higher handgrip strength and ADL-score, which has already been observed in previous studies (HOUSTON ET AL. 2007, BISCHOFF-FERRARI ET AL. 2004). Comparable with a vicious circle, nursing home residents show a higher risk of low vitamin D levels due to lower functional ability, which may influence their time spent outside vice versa; because UV-light is necessary for vitamin D synthesis, this might again reinforce the low vitamin D level and therefore contribute to a decline in muscle function (HOLICK 1998). Additionally, the concentration of 7-dehydrocholesterol, the precursor of vitamin D_3 in the skin, decreases with age and therefore reinforces low vitamin D concentrations in blood as well (HOLICK AND CHEN 2008).

In other studies, different mean vitamin D levels were observed in the annual comparison due to this seasonal dependency of ultraviolet radiation (PEREZ-LLAMAS ET AL. 2008). The present nursing home residents also showed a significant decline in vitamin D levels within one year, which might either be explained by a decline in functionality or a decline in reserves. Seasonal influences can be disregarded in this case due to the continuous process of blood withdrawals in all participants and the individual distance of 12 months.

The association of lower vitamin D levels with higher mortality rates (VISSER ET AL. 2006, ZITTERMANN ET AL. 2009) has been confirmed by the present study (see figure VIII), which might be explained by several reasons. It has been shown that low vitamin D levels are associated with two aspects. First, lower functionality may increase the risk for fractures due to falls, representing a predictor of a bad outcome. Secondly, there is an association of vitamin D deficiency and several chronic morbidities such as cardiovascular diseases, osteoporosis, and diabetes (BISCHOFF-FERRARI ET AL. 2004, BISCHOFF-FERRARI ET AL. 2008, KILKKINEN ET AL. 2009, HOLICK 2004, SCRAGG ET AL. 2004), which also increases the risk of death. In addition to the high prevalence of chronic diseases in nursing home residents, another fact may explain the association between low vitamin D levels and mortality. During the terminal phase of life, elderly people often show a low nutritional intake and relevant weight loss, resulting in an exhaustion of vitamin reserves. Furthermore, nursing home residents are characterized on all accounts by higher mortality compared with community-living persons due to the high age, the high prevalence of chronic diseases as well as highly relevant cognitive and physical deficits.

Compared to the present study, higher retinol levels and a lower prevalence of retinol deficiency have been shown in healthy adults (GARRY ET AL. 1987, HESEKER ET AL. 1992), free-living elderly volunteers (PANEMANGALORE AND LEE 1992) and in older frail and non-frail community-dwelling women (SEMBA ET AL. 2006). The present results reveal retinol levels that are similar to those described for very old, independently living older people in Germany (VOLKERT ET AL. 1992). One hypothesis is that the high prevalence of retinol deficiency indicates a low intake of fresh fruit and vegetables, which is a typical problem in nursing homes, which might be explained by the one-sided preference of older people regarding food choice or the presence of chewing and swallowing problems, especially with hard and fresh meals. Additionally, fresh vegetables are more expensive for the nursing homes and handling is more time-intensive, as it cannot be stored over a long period. This hypothesis may also explain the lower prevalence of retinol deficiency shown in several French nursing homes, where only 10.8% of women and 16.1% of men showed levels below 161 µg/l (corresponds to 20.2% in the present study using the same cut-off) (MONGET ET AL. 1996), possibly caused by a more Mediterranean food pattern and different food habits in France, which might be more rich in fresh fruit, vegetables and giblets.

The observed differences between the prevalence of low retinol levels in men and women in the present study could also result from greater awareness of women to consume more fresh fruit and vegetables, often displaying a greater health consciousness. However, this hypothesis was not confirmed in French nursing home residents with higher prevalence of retinol deficiency in women (MONGET ET AL. 1996). Furthermore, our results show that higher retinol and folate levels were associated with functional parameters, which strengthens the hypothesis that a good nutritional situation is associated with higher physical performance.

To interpret the albumin status, age-related serum levels within less than 3.0 and less than 3.4 g/dl were used as age-adjusted cut-offs for a low status, which was present in 26% of the residents (see table IX). In institutionalized elderly a lower level of albumin has been observed than in their free-living counterparts (SAHYOUN ET AL. 1988). When 3.5 g/dl was used as a cut-off point, Pauly and co-workers found prevalence rates between < 5% and 58% in nursing home residents worldwide (PAULY ET AL. 2007). In the present study, albumin was measured as an indicator of the protein status. In addition to the nutritional status of the patient, albumin levels are influenced by inflammatory processes, as protein levels decrease in case of acute disease (BAUER ET AL. 2006). It has also been shown that low serum albumin levels were associated with an increased risk of infection, decubitus ulcers, prolonged nursing home stays and mortality (MORLEY AND SILVER 1995). Even though albumin is discussed as rather less appropriate predictor for protein status in the literature, analysis showed that it was positively associated with handgrip strength and ADL-score as functional indicators in the present study. Apart from the good nutritional status indicated by most of the measured nutrients, as well as by the calculated mean of BMI, protein seems to be one of the most problematic nutrients in this setting, as underlined by the observed rather low medium values.

Data on ß-carotene in nursing home residents are scarce; present studies in community-dwelling elderly, focusing the intake of ß-carotene or total carotenoid plasma level, i.e. in the SENECA study, found plasma levels between 0.28 and 0.69 µmol/l in European elderly (BUIJSSE ET AL. 2005). In the present study, 9.7% of the residents showed a deficiency of ß-carotene with levels below 0.18 µmol/l (see table IX). Due to the different population, this was, as expected, a higher rate than described for healthy adults (6.6%) (HESEKER ET AL. 1992).

Vitamin B_{12} deficiency is highly prevalent in elderly people. Multimedication is regarded as one main contributing factor for B_{12} deficiency in older people, due to a decreased absorption of this micronutrient emerging from the complex absorption process, in which the intrinsic factor of the gastric acid is included (STROEHLE ET AL. 2004). In the present study, 8.6% of the residents showed a low B_{12} level (see table IX), which is higher than the prevalence of 3%, which was found in a healthy older population. In this study, a higher cut-off point of approximately 162 pmol/l was used (GARRY ET AL. 1984). The mean level was comparable to free-living adults (NG ET AL. 2009) but lower than the mean level of healthy adults in the VERA-study (HESEKER ET AL. 1992). Baik and Russell reported prevalence rates between 3% and 40.5% in elderly across all settings, depending on the applied diagnostic criteria (BAIK AND RUSSELL 1999). In the literature, vitamin B_{12} deficiency is associated with an increased risk of neurodegenerative diseases (ALLEN ET AL. 1998), as well as pernicious anemia (BAIK AND RUSSELL 1999). Also it was shown that a replacement of B_{12} can increase cognitive function (VAN DYCK ET AL. 2009). The discussion on the cut-off value for B_{12} deficiency is ongoing; it was reported that a cut-off value of 200 pg/ml might be too low and may underestimate the B_{12} deficiency frequency. With a cut-off value of 350 pg/ml (258 pmol/l), as used in the Framingham study, which included free-living elderly aged 67 to 96 years, deficiency was determined for 40.5% (BAIK AND RUSSELL 1999). By using the lower cut-off value of 148 pmol/l, the prevalence rate decreased to 5.3%. In a mixed population of nursing home residents and free-living elderly, a prevalence of 20% was shown, using a cut-off rate of <150 pmol/l. However, the sub-group of nursing home residents showed a higher prevalence of deficiency than the group of free-living elderly (BATES ET AL. 2003). A prevalence of 8.6% of B_{12} deficiency was shown in the present study using a cut-off point of 141 pmol/l. By using a cut-off value similar to a study in Spanish nursing home residents ($\leq$ 200 pg/ml), prevalence increased to 9.2% in the present study, which was still lower than 15.8% as described for the Spanish nursing home population (GONZALES-GROSS ET AL. 2007). A higher prevalence of B_{12} deficiency in nursing home residents might be explained by the high consumption of drugs in this population, being characterized by chronic diseases, as confirmed in the present study.

Folate deficiency was lower (6.5%) in the present nursing home residents than in Dutch residents (28%) (LOEWIK ET AL. 1992) and obviously higher in comparison to free-living elderly with no deficiency, however, here the cut-off value was set lower (SCHLETTWEIN–GSELL ET AL. 1999). The measured mean folate level was higher than previously shown in nursing home residents (WOUTERS-WESSELING ET AL. 2002, ALLSUP ET AL. 2004). Spanish nursing home residents showed comparable (GONZALEZ-GROSS ET AL. 2007) and US residents and US free-living elderly showed higher folate levels (SAHYOUN ET AL. 1988, SEMBA ET AL. 2006). German adults from the VERA study showed similar levels (HESEKER ET AL. 1992). As folate intake is often described as insufficient in Europe, the low prevalence of folate deficiency in the present study can be regarded as delectable.

The α-tocopherol levels were comparably high to those in community-dwelling elderly (CESARI ET AL. 2004, BLE ET AL. 2006, BUJSSE ET AL. 2005) and adults (HESEKER ET AL. 1992), and even higher than in free-living elderly Americans (PANEMANGALORE AND

LEE 1992) and moderately to severe disabled community-dwelling women (SEMBA ET AL. 2006). Deficiency prevalence was comparable to French nursing home residents showing adequate levels of α-tocopherol (MONGET ET AL. 1996). It has been described that a balanced diet offers a sufficient amount of 10-15 mg/d vitamin E when vegetable oils are consumed (BIESALSKI ET AL. 1995). Unfortunately, the nutritional intake was not assessed in the present study, but it may be presumed that the intake of vegetable oil applies to German food habits also in frail elderly. Fortunately, only one resident showed a low cholesterol/α-tocopherol ratio. This data was confirmed by nursing home residents in France (MONGET ET AL. 1996).

Enteral feeding

The prevalence of PEG was relatively low (5.5%) and slightly lower than present in German nursing homes with 6.6% (WIRTH ET AL. 2009) and the European mean of 5.9% detected in the NutritionDay in nursing homes in 2007 (VALENTINI ET AL. 2009). Data on the nutrient blood levels of tube-fed nursing home residents are scarce. In the present study, significantly higher values of vitamin D and folate have been shown in these residents. The tocopherol/cholesterol ratio was better than in residents with normal food, too. A significantly lower cholesterol level was found in nasogastric-fed patients with advanced dementia in the community (ALVAREZ-FERNÁNDEZ ET AL. 2005). While the present study did not show any significant differences between the albumin levels, Breslow and co-workers found a significantly higher albumin level of 37 g/l in non-tube-fed nursing home residents compared with tube-fed patients (33 g/l) (BRESLOW ET AL. 1991). In a Cochrane Collaboration review, data in this regard were inconsistent (SAMPSON ET AL. 2009). Most of the residents showing severe chewing or swallowing difficulties in the present study were fed by PEG. Enteral nutrition aims to assure an adequate supply of all nutrients in these residents, which is confirmed by the present data. Compared with cognitive impaired non-tube fed residents, the problem of an insufficient nutritional intake is solved thereby. Although a better nutritional status, which should be the target of enteral feeding, seems to be associated with survival, there was no significant difference of mortality in those two groups in the present study. Alvarez-Fernández found an increased relative risk for mortality in nasogastric-fed patients with advanced dementia (ALVAREZ-FERNÁNDEZ ET AL. 2005). However, the ethical discussion on the effect of enteral nutrition on quality of life, functionality and mortality in demented patients is ongoing (SAMPSON ET AL. 2009).

Follow-up blood levels

Vitamin D and retinol level significantly decreased within one year of observation while all other nutrient blood levels remained stable. In addition to the above-mentioned hypotheses on the decline of vitamin D levels, the drop of retinol may also be explained by the decline in the functional and cognitive ability in this population, possibly being associated with one-sided nutrition, poor in retinol. Comparable data are not yet available.

Blood markers and mortality

Nutrient levels of survivors showed only a tendency to be higher than in residents who deceased during the study, except for the ß-carotene and vitamin B_{12}. Studies considering nutrient status and survival were published for the risk of cancer in adults (STAEHELIN ET AL. 1991) and for non-institutionalized elderly (SAHYOUN ET AL. 1996) but not in nursing home residents yet, due to the lack of longitudinal studies in this setting. One hypothesis for this result is, on the one hand, the association of a better nutritional situation in elderly people with survival, which has been shown in several studies before (DE GROOT AND VAN STAVEREN 2002, CHAN ET AL. 2010, SAHYOUN ET AL. 1996). On the other hand, low nutrient levels may be a consequence of low nutritional intake, which often leads to death, or displays a precursor of death. Due to the non-significant results of the present study in this regard, it may be stated that existing nutrient resources, especially in lipid-soluble vitamins and albumin, which can be stored for a long period, lead to only a trend between nutrient status of survivors and deceased being shown in this population.

Blood level and functionality

The association of vitamin D and albumin levels with higher functional abilities have already been explained by the present data as aforementioned as well as in several studies. Significant correlations between retinol level and ADL score and the folate level and gait speed have not yet been investigated and require further research in this regard.

Conclusion

In the present study an adequate mean level of all analyzed nutrients except for vitamin D was shown. The prevalence of blood marker deficiency was highest for vitamin D, retinol and albumin. In comparison to most community living elderly, the prevalence of deficiency of nutritional blood markers was higher in nursing home residents. Malnutrition is often associated with frailty and increased dependency, which is highly present in nursing home residents. This fact may also be the reason for the significant decline of several specific blood markers within one year of follow-up.

Percutaneous endoscopic gastrostomy fed residents showed significant higher levels of vitamin D- and folate as well as a higher α-tocopherol/cholesterol ratio. With artificial nutritional support an adequate supply of macro- and micronutrients in elderly with cognitive deficits or with chewing or swallowing difficulties seems to be easier to assure. Nevertheless, the ethical discussion with regard to enteral feeding in the elderly population has to be taken into account.

In the present study, associations between vitamin D, retinol, folate and albumin level and parameters of functionality have been shown. The association between vitamin D and function has already been observed in several studies and is explicable firstly, by the positive influence from vitamin D on muscle tissue and secondly, by the activated synthesis of vitamin D in skin by UV-light, which might only concern mobile residents.

Correlations between the retinol and folate level and functional parameters might be explained by a generally better nutritional status in the group of elderly without highly relevant functional deficits. Nevertheless, this field requires further investigation.

The association between mortality and low nutrient blood levels could only be confirmed with regard to vitamin D level. Due to the lack of longitudinal studies investigating nursing home residents, no comparable data are available at this point.

One hypothesis for this result is on the one hand the association of a better nutritional situation in elderly people with survival, which has been shown in several studies before. On the other hand, low nutrient levels may be a consequence of low nutritional intake, which often leads to death, or displays a precursor of death. Long ranged nutrient resources, especially of lipid-soluble vitamins and albumin may have resulted in the non-significant differences regarding prevalence of nutrient deficiencies of survivors and deceased in the present study.

References III

ALLEN RH, STABLER SP, LINDENBAUM J. Relevance of vitamins, homocysteine and other metabolites in neuropsychiatric disorders. *Eur J Pediatr.* 1998;157(2):122-6.

ALLSUP SJ, SHENKIN A, PATH FRC, GOSNEY MA, TAYLOR S, TAYLOR W, HAMMOND M, ZAMBON MC. Can a Short Period of Micronutrient Supplementation in Older Institutionalized People Improve Response to Influenza Vaccine? A Randomized, Controlled Trial. *J Am Geriatr Soc.* 2004;52:20-24.

ALVAREZ-FERNÁNDEZ B, GARCÍA-ORDONEZ MA, MARTÍNEZ-MANZANARES C, GÓMEZ-HUELGAS R. Survival of a cohort of elderly patients with advanced dementia: nasogastric tube feeding as a risk factor for mortality. *Int J Geriatr Psychiatry* 2005;20:363-370.

BAIK HW, RUSSELL RM. B_{12} deficiency in the elderly. *Annu Rev Nutr.* 1999;19:357-77.

BARTALI B, SEMBA RD, FRONGILLO EA, VARADHAN R, RICKS MO, BLAUM CS, FERRUCCI L, JM, FRIED LP. Low Micronutrient Levels as a Predictor of Incident Disability in Older Women. *Arch Intern Med.* 2006;166:2335-2340.

BARTALI B, FRONGILLO EA, GURALNIK JM, STIPANUK MH, ALLORE HC, CHERUBINI A, BANDINELLI S, FERRUCCI L, GILL TM. Serum Micronutrient Concentrations and Decline in Physical Function Among Older Persons. *J Am Med Assoc.* 2008;299(3):308-315.

BASHA B, RAO DS, HAN ZH, PARFITT AM. Osteomalacia due to vitamin D depletion: a neglected consequence of intestinal malabsorption. *Am J Med.* 2000;108(4):296-300.

BATES CJ, SCHNEEDE J, MISHRA G, PRENTICE A, MANSOOR MA. Relationship between methylmalonic acid, homocysteine, vitamin B_{12} intake and status and socio-economic indices, in a subset of participants in the British National Diet and Nutrition Survey of people aged 65 y and over. *Eur J Clin Nutr.* 2003;57:349-357.

BAUER JM, VOLKERT D, WIRTH R, VELLAS B, THOMAS D, KONDRUP J, PIRLICH M, WERNER HJ, SIEBER CC. Diagnostik der Mangelernährung des älteren Menschen. *Dtsch Med Wochenschr.* 2006;131:223-227.

BAUER JM, KAISER M, ANTHONY P, GUIGOZ Y, SIEBER CC. The Mini Nutritional Assessment-Its History, Today's Practice, and Future Perspectives. *Nutr Clin Pract. 2008;23(4):388-96.*

BIESALSKI HK, BÖHLES H, ESTERBAUER H, FÜRST P, GEY KF, KASPER H, SIES H, WEISBURGER J, HUNDSDÖRFER G. Antioxidative Vitamine in der Prävention. *Deutsches Ärzteblatt 1995;92:A-1316-1231.*

BISCHOFF-FERRARI HA, GIOVANNUCCI E, WILLETT WC, DIETRICH T, DAWSON-HUGHES B. Estimation of optimal serum concentration of 25-hydroxyvitamin D for multiple health outcomes. *Am J Clin Nutr. 2006;84:18-28.*

BISCHOFF-FERRARI HA, DIETRICH T, ORAV EJ, HU FB, ZHANG Y, KARLSON EW, DAWSON-HUGHES B. Higher 25-hydroxyvitamin D concentrations are associated with better lower-extremity function in both active and inactive persons aged $\geq$ 60 y. *Am J Clin Nutr. 2004;80:752-758.*

BISCHOFF HA, STAHELIN HB, URSCHELER N, EHRSAM R, VONTHEIN R, PERRIG-CHIELLO P, TYNDALL A, THEILER R. Muscle Strength in the Elderly: Its Relation to Vitamin D Metabolites. *Arch Phy Med Rehabil. 1999;80:54-58.*

BJOERKEGREN K, SVAERDSUDD K. Serum cobalamin, folate, methylmalonic acid and total homocysteine as vitamin B12 and folate tissue deficiency markers amongst elderly Swedes – a population-based study. *J Intern Med. 2001;249:423-432.*

BLE A, CHERUBINI A, VOLPATO S, BARTALI B, WALSTON JD, WINDHAM BG, BANDINELLI S, LAURETANI F, GURALNIK JM, FERRUCCI L. Lower plasma Vitamin E Levels Are Associated With the Frailty Syndrome: The InCHIANTI Study. *J Gerontol. 2006;61(3):278-283.*

BRESLOW RA, HALLFRISCH J, GOLDBERG AP. Malnutrition in Tubefed Nursing Home Patients With Pressure Sores. *J Parenter Enteral Nutr. 1991;15(6):663-668.*

BROE KE, CHEN TC, WEINBERG J, BISCHOFF-FERRARI HA, HOLICK MF, KIEL DP. A Higher Dose of Vitamin D Reduces the Risk of Falls in Nursing Home Residents: A Randomized, Multiple-Dose Study. *J Am Geriatr Soc. 2007;55:243-239.*

BROWNIE S. Why are elderly individuals at risk of nutritional deficiency? *Int J Nurs Pract. 2006;12:110-118.*

BUIJSSE B, FESKENS EJM, SCHLETTWEIN-GSELL D, FERRY M, KOK FJ, KROMHOUT D, DE GROOT LCPGM FOR THE SENECA INVESTIGATORS. Plasma carotene and α-tocopherol in relation to 10-y all-cause and caise-specific mortality in European elderly: the Survey in Europe on Nutrition and the Elderly, a Concerted Action (SENECA). *Am J Clin Nutr. 2005;82:879-886.*

CESARI M, PAHOR M, BARTALI B, CHERUBINI A, PENNINX B, WILLIAMS GR, ATKINSON H, MARTIN A, GURALNIK JM, FERRUCCI L. Antioxidants and physical performance in elderly persons: the Invecchiare in Chianti (InCHIANTI) study. *Am J Clin Nutr. 2004;79:289-294.*

CHAN M, LIM YP, ERNEST A, TAN TL. Nutritional assessment in an Asian nursing home and its association with mortality. *J Nutr Health Aging 2010;14(1):23-8.*

CHUMLEA W, ROCHE A, STEINBAUGH M: estimating stature from knee height for persons 60-90 years of age. *J Am Geriatr Soc. 1985;33:116-120.*

CHUMLEA WW, GUO S, WHOLIHAN K, ET AL. Stature predictions equations for elderly non-Hispanic white, non-Hispanic black and Mexican American persons developed from NHANES-III data. *J Amer dietet Assoc. 1998;98:137-142.*

D-A-CH Referenzwerte Deutsche Gesellschaft für Ernährung, Österreichische Gesellschaft für Ernährung, Schweizerische Gesellschaft für Ernährungsforschung, Schweizerische Vereinigung für Ernährung. Referenzwerte für die Nährstoffzufuhr. 1. Auflage. Umschau/ Braus-Verlag, Frankfurt/Main, 2000.

DE GROOT CPGM, VAN STAVEREN WA. Undernutrition in the European SENECA studies. *Clin Geriatr Med. 2002;18:699-708.*

DREWNOWSKI A, SHULTZ JM. Impact of aging on eating behaviors, food choices, nutrition, and health status. *J Nutr Health Aging 2001;5(2):75-9.*

FLETCHER AE, BREEZE E, SHETTY PS. Antioxidant vitamins and mortality in older persons: findings from the nutrition add-on study to the Medical Research Council Trail of Assessment and Management of Older People in the Community. *Am J Clin Nutr. 2003;78:999-1010.*

FOLSTEIN MF, FOLSTEIN S, MCHUGH PR: Mini Mental State: a practical method for grading cognitive state of patients for the clinician. *J Psychiatr Res. 1975;12:189-198*

GARRY PJ, GOODWIN JS, HUNT WC. Folate and vitamin B_{12} status in a healthy elderly population. *J Am Geriatr Soc. 1984;32(10):719-26.*

GARRY PJ, HUNT WC, BANDROFCHAK JL, VANDERJAGT D, GODDWIN JS. Vitamin A intake and plasma retinol levels in healthy elderly men and women. *Am J Clin Nutr. 1987;46:989-994.*

GONZALEZ-GROSS M, SOLA R, ALBERS U, BARRIOS L, ALDER M, CASTILLO ML, PIETRZIK K. B-Vitamins and Homocysteine in Spanish Institutionalized Elderly. *Int J Vitam Nutr Res. 2007;77(1):22-33.*

GUIGOZ Y, VELLAS B, GARRY PJ: Mini Nutritional Assessment: a practical assessment tool for grading the nutritional state of elderly patients. *Facts Res Gerontol. 1994;(2):15-60.*

GUIGOZ Y, VELLAS B, GARRY PJ: Assessing the Nutritional Status of the elderly. The Mini Nutritional Assessment as Part of the Geriatric Evaluation. *Nutrition reviews 1996;54:59-65.*

HARRILL I, CERVONE N. Vitamin Status of older women. *Am J Clin Nutr. 1977;30:431-440.*

HARRIS SS, DAWSON-HUGHES B. Plasma vitamin D and 25OHD responses of young and old men to supplementation with vitamin D3. *J Am Coll Nutr. 2002;21:357-62.*

HESEKER H, SCHNEIDER R, MOCH KJ, KOHLMEIER M, KÜBLER W. Vitaminversorgung Erwachsener in der Bundesrepublik Deutschland. In: Kohlmeier M (ed): *VERA-Schriftenreihe, vol IV. Wissenschaftlicher Fachverlag Dr. Fleck, Niederkleen, 1992:110ff.*

HIMENO M, TSUGAWA N, KUWABARA A, FUJII M, KAWAI N, KATO Y, KIHARA N, TOYODA T. KISHIMOTO M, OGAWA Y, KIDO S, NOIKE T, OKANO T, TANAKA K. Effect of vitamin D supplementation in the institutionalized elderly. *J Bone Miner Metab. 2009;27:733–737.*

HOLICK MF, CHEN TC. Vitamin D deficiency: a worldwide problem with health consequences. *Am J Clin Nutr. 2008;87(suppl):1080S-1086S.*

HOLICK MF. Vitamin D Deficiency. *N Engl J Med. 2007;357:266-281.*

HOLICK MF. Sunlight and vitamin D for bone health and prevention of autoimmune diseases, cancers, and cardiovascular disease. *Am J Clin Nutr. 2004;80 (suppl):1678S– 88S.*

HOLICK MF. Vitamin D requirements for humans of all ages: new increased requirements for women and men 50 years and older. *Osteoporos Int. 1998;8(2):24-29.*

HOUSTON DK, CESARI M, FERRUCCI L, CHERUBINI A, MAGGIO D, BARTALI B, JOHNSON MA, SCHWARTZ GG, KRITCHEVSKY SB. Association Between Vitamin D Status and Physical Performance: The InCHIANTI Study. *J Gerontol. 2007;62(4):440-446.*

JOHNSON AM, GUDER WG. ALBUMIN. In: Ritchie RF, Novolotskaia O, eds. Serum proteins in clinical medicine. *Scarborough: Foundation for Blood Research, 1996;6.00:1-10.*

KARG G, GEDRICH K. Neuauswertung der Nationalen Verzehrsstudie (1985.1989). In: *Ernährungsbericht 1996. (Deutsche Gesellschaft fuer Ernaehrung, ed.). Druckerei Henrich, Frankfurt/Main:37-53.*

KILKKINEN A, KNEKT P, ARO A, RISSANEN H, MARNIEMI J, HELIÖVAARA M, IMPIVAARA O, REUNANEN A. Vitamin D status and the risk of cardiovascular disease death. *Am J Epidemiol. 2009;170(8):1032-9. Epub 2009 Sep 17.*

KUWABARA A, TSUGAWA N,TANAKA K, FUJII M, KAWAI M, MUKAE S, KATO Y, KOJIMA Y, TAKAHASHI K, KAZUMASA O, KAGAWA R, INOUE A, NOIKE T, KIDO S, OKANO T. Improvement of Vitamin D status in Japanese institutionalized Elderly by Supplementation with 800 IU of Vitamin D_3. *J Nutr Sci Vitaminol. 2009;55:453-458.*

LESHER EL, BERRYHILL JS: Validation of the Geriatric Depression Scale-short form among inpatients. *J Clin Psychol. 1994;50:256-60.*

LIPS P, WIERSINGA A, VAN GINKEL FC, JONGEN MJ, NETELENBOS JC, HACKENG WH, DELMAS PD, VAN DER VIJGH WJ. The effect of vitamin D supplementation on vitamin D status and parathyroid function in elderly subjects. *J Clin Endocrinol Metab. 1988;67:644-50.*

LIPS M ET AL. Vitamin D status and muscoloskeletal Health in the Longitudinal Aging Stud Amsterdam (LASA); Different Thresholds for Different Outcomes. *JBMR 2006;21(1):F302.*

LIU BA, MCGEER A, MCARTHUR MA, SIMOR AE, AGHDASSI E, DAVIS L, ALLARD JP. Effect of Multivitamin and Mineral Supplementation on Episodes of Infection in Nursing Home Residents: A Randomized, Placebo-controlled Study. *J Am Geriatr Soc. 2007;55:35-42.*

LOEWIK MR, VAN DEN BERG H, SCHRIJVER J, ODINK J, WEDEL M, VAN HOUTEN P. Marginal nutritional status among institutionalized elderly women as compared to those living more independently (Dutch Nutrition Surveillance System). *J Am Coll Nutr. 1992;11(6):673-681.*

MAHONEY FI, BARTHEL DW: Functional Evaluation: The Barthel Index. *Maryland State Medical Journal 1965;14: 61-65.*

MINI NUTRITIONAL ASSESSMENT: *www.mna-elderly.com 03.12.2009*

MONGET AL, GALAN P, PREZIOSI P, KELLER H, BOURGEOIS C, ARNAUD J, FAVIER A, HERCBERG S AND THE GERIATRIE / MIN. VIT. AOX NETWORK. Micronutrient Status in Elderly people. *Internat J Vit Nutr Res. 1996:71-76.*

MOREIRA-PFRIMER L, PEDROSA MAC, TEIXEIRA L, LAZARETTI-CASTRO M. Treatment of Vitamin D Deficiency Increases Lower Limb Muscle Strength in Institutionalized Older People Independently of Regular Physical Activity: A Randomized Double-Blind Controlled Trial. *Ann Nutr Metab. 2009;54:291-300.*

MORLEY JE. Anorexia of aging: physiologic and pathologic. *Am J Clin Nutr 1997;66:760-773.*

MORLEY JE, SILVER AJ. Nutritional Issues in Nursing Home Care. *Ann Intern Med 1995;123(11): 850-859.*

MORRIS MC, EVANS DA, BIENIAS JL, TANGNEY CC, WILSON RS. Vitamin E and cognitive Decline in Older Persons. *Arch Neurol. 2002;59:1125-1132.*

MORRISSEY PA, SHEEHY PJ, GAYNOR P. Vitamin E. *Int J Vitam Nutr Res. 1993;63(4):260-4.*

NG TP, FENG L, NITI M, KUA EH, YAP KB. Folate, Vitamin B12, Homocysteine, and depressive Symptoms in a Population Sample of Older Chinese Adults. *J Am Geriatr Soc. 2009;57:871-876.*

PANEMANGALORE M, LEE CJ. Evaluation of the Indices of Retinol and α-Tocopherol Status in Free-Living Elderly. *J Gerontol. 1992;47(3):B98-104.*

PAPAPETROU PD, TRIANTAFYLLOPOULOU M, KORAKOVOUNI A. Severe vitamin D deficiency in the institutionalized elderly. *J Endocrinol Invest. 2008;31(9):784-7.*

PAULY L, STEHLE P, VOLKERT D. Nutritional situation of elderly nursing home residents. *Z Gerontol Geriat. 2007;40:1-10.*

PEACOCK M. Osteomalacia and rickets. In: *Nordin BEC, Need AG, Morris HA, eds. Metabolic bone and stone disease. Edinburgh: Churchill Livingstone, 1993:83-108.*

PÉREZ-LLAMAS F, LOPEZ-CONTRERAS MJ, BLANCO MJ, LÓPEZ-AZORÍN F, ZAMORA S, MOREIRAS O. Seemingly paradoxical seasonal influences on vitamin D status in nursing-home elderly people from a Mediterranean area. *Nutrition* 2008;24:414-420.

SAMPSON EL, CANDY B, JONES L. Enteral tube feeding for older people with advanced dementia (review). *The Cochrane Collaboration 2009. Published by John Wiley & Sons, Ltd.1-25.*

SAHYOUN NR, JACQUES PF, RUSSELL RM. Carotinoids, Vitamin C and E, and Mortality in an Elderly Population. *Am J Epidemiol.* 1996;144(5):501-511.

SAHYOUN NR, OTRADOVEC CL, HARTZ SC, JACOB RA, PETERS H, RUSSELL RM, MCGANDY RB. Dietary intakes and biochemical indicators of nutritional status in an elderly, institutionalized poulation. *Am J Clin Nutr.* 1988;47:524-533.

SCHLETTWEIN-GSELL, DECARLI B, AMORIM CRUZ JA, HALLER J, DE GROOT C.PGM, VAN STAVEREN WA. Nährstoffaufnahme bei gesunden Betagten. *Z Gerontol Geriat.* 1999;32(1): I/1–I/6.

SCRAGG R, SOWERS M, BELL C. Third National Health and Nutrition Examination Survey. Serum 25-hydroxyvitamin D, diabetes, and ethnicity in the Third National Health and Nutrition Examination Survey. *Diabetes Care* 2004;27(12):2813-8.

SEMBA RD, BARTALI B, ZHOU J, BLAUM C, KO C-W, FRIED LP. Low Serum Micronutrient Concentrations Predict Frailty Among Older Women Living in the Community. *J Gerontol.* 2006;61(6):594-599.

SHEIK JL, YESAVAGE JA. Geriatric depression scale (GDS): recent evidence and development of a shorter version. *Clin Gerontol.* 1986;37:819–820.

STAEHELIN HB, GEY KF, EICHHOLZER M, LÜDIN E, BERNASCONI F, THURNEYSEN J, BRUBACHER G. Plasma antioxidant vitamins and subsequent cancer mortality in the 12-year follow-up of the prospective Basel Study. *Am J Epidemiol.* 1991;133(8):766-75.

STOEHLE A, WOLTER M, HAHN A. Vitamin B12-Mangel im höheren Lebensalter. *E-Umschau* 2004;51(3):90-96.

VALENTINI L, SCHINDLER K, SCHLAFFER R, BUCHER, H, MOUHIEDDINE M, STEININGER K, TRIPAMER, J, HANDSCHUH M, SCHUH C, VOLKERT D, LOCHS, H, SIEBER CC, HIESMAYR M: The first nutritionDay in nursing homes: participation may improve malnutrition awareness. *Clin Nutr.* 2009; 28: 109-116.

VAN DYCK CH, LYNESS JM, ROHRBAUGH RM, SIEGAL AP. Cognitive and psychiatric effects of vitamin B12 replacement in dementia with low serum B_{12} levels: a nursing home study. *Int Psychogeriatr. 2009;21(1):138–147.*

VISSER M, DEEG DJH, PUTS MTE, SEIDELL JC, LIPS P. Low serum concentrations of 25-hydroxyvitamin D in older persons and the risk of nursing home admission. *Am J Clin Nutr. 2006;84:616-622.*

VOLKERT D, FRAUENRATH C, MICOL W, KRUSE W, OSTER P, SCHLIERF G. Nutritional status of the very old: anthropometric and biochemical findings in apparently healthy women in old's people's home. *Aging 1992;4(1):21-28.*

VOLKERT D, STEHLE P. Vitamin Status of Elderly People in Germany. *Int J Vitam Nutr Res. 1999;69(3):154-159.*

VUILLEUMIER J-P, KELLER HE, GYSEL D, HUNZIKER F. Clinical Chemical Methods for the Routine Assessment of the Vitamin Status in Human Populations. *Internat J Vit Nutr Res. 1983;53:265-272.*

WIRTH R, BAUER JM, WILLSCHREI HP, VOLKERT D, SIEBER CC. Prevalence of percutanous Endoscopic Gastrostomy in Nursing Home residents – A Nationwide Survey in Germany. *Gerontology 2009 2009;11, Epub ahead of print.*

WOUTERS-WESSELING W, WOUTERS AEJ, KLEIJER CN, BINDELS JG, DE GROOT CPGM, VAN STAVEREN WA. Study on the effect of a liquid nutrition supplement on the nutritional status of psycho-geriatric nursing home patients. *Eur J Clin Nutr. 2002;56:245-251.*

WRIGHT JD, BIALOSTOSKY K, GUNTER EW, CARROLL MD, NAJJAR MF, BOWMAN BA, JOHNSON CL. Blood folate and vitamin B12: United States, 1988-94. *Vital Health Stat. 1998;11(243):1-78.*

ZITTERMANN A. Vitamin D and diesease prevention with special reference to cardiovascular disease. *Prog Biophys Mol Biol. 2006;92(1):39-48.*

ZITTERMANN A, GUMMERT JF, BÖRGERMANN J. Vitamin D deficiency and mortality. *Curr Opin Clin Nutr Metab Care 2009;12(6):634-9.*

CHAPTER FOUR

Functionality and Mortality in Obese Nursing Home Residents –
An Example of 'Risk Factor Paradox'?

Kaiser et al., published in J Am Med Dir Assoc. 2010;11(6):428-35

Abstract

Background: While the percentage of obese nursing home residents is increasing, few longitudinal studies have reported on functionality and mortality in this subpopulation. The aim of the present study was to explore functionality and mortality in obese nursing home residents during a one-year follow-up and to compare these results with those of residents within the normal and low body mass index (BMI) range. Methods: Two hundred residents (147 female, 53 male, mean age 85.6±7.8 years) from two Nuremberg nursing homes were included. Body weight and height were measured in all participants. BMI was calculated and categorized as low (<20 kg/m²), normal (20-30 kg/m²) and high (>30 kg/m²). Handgrip strength, timed 'up and go' test and Barthel's Activities of Daily Living were applied as functional parameters. All measurements were done at baseline and after a one-year follow-up. Results: At baseline the prevalence of obesity was 23.5%, while low BMI values were present in 8.5% of the residents. After one year, there was no significant decline of functionality in the obese group, while functional parameters deteriorated significantly in study participants with normal BMI. One-year mortality was lowest in the obese (12.8%), with no deaths in residents with BMI ≥35 kg/m². Mortality was highest in residents with low BMI (58.8%). Conclusion: In nursing home residents obesity is associated with increased survival and stable functionality. These observations may therefore be regarded as an expression of 'risk factor paradox' in this specific population of older individuals.

Introduction

In most western societies, the prevalence of obesity in older persons has been increasing constantly in past decades. A recent study on newly admitted nursing home residents reported that the prevalence of obesity rose from 15% to more than 25% between 1992 and 2002 [1]. Bradway observed a predominance of studies focusing on community-dwelling obese elderly and a lack of surveys regarding obese nursing home residents [2]. A negative association between body weight and functionality in community-dwelling older persons or newly admitted nursing home residents was found in several studies [3-11].

To our knowledge, corresponding data on nutritional status, functional parameters for nursing home residents have not yet been published and data on mortality in obese nursing home residents are still scarce.

The association between high Body Mass Index (BMI) and mortality in older persons in general has been analyzed in numerous studies. While some found an increased risk of mortality among community-living obese elderly compared to those with normal weight [12,13], other authors observed a decreased mortality risk in those with high BMI [14-16] or at least no increased risk [17]. Data on the relationship between high BMI and mortality in nursing home residents have also been inconsistent [18,19].

As information on functionality and mortality in nursing home residents is highly relevant for the judgment of the level of care that society will have to face in future decades it is important to provide additional data in this field.

The aim of the present study was to explore the association of obesity with functionality and mortality in nursing home residents during a one-year follow-up.

Methods

All residents of two communal nursing homes in Nuremberg, Germany, were approached to participate in the present study from June 2007 until December 2008. Residents aged below 65 years and in palliative care with a very limited life expectancy were excluded. Informed consent was obtained from all participating residents or their legal proxies. The study protocol was approved by the ethics committees of the Friedrich-Alexander-University of Erlangen-Nuremberg, Germany, and the Rheinische Friedrich-Wilhelms-University of Bonn, Germany.

Characteristics

Cognitive status was evaluated by the Mini Mental State Examination (MMSE) [20]. Emotional status was assessed using the 15-item Geriatric Depression Scale (GDS), as validated by Lesher and Berryhill [21]. The number of drugs taken was collected from the residents' files.

Nutritional status

The nutritional status was evaluated by the Mini Nutritional Assessment® (MNA [22]), a screening tool for malnutrition which was specifically developed for use in the elderly [23-25]. With the exception of its anthropometric items, the MNA was completed by the nursing staff.

The following anthropometric measurements were performed in all participants: weight, knee height, mid-arm circumference, waist circumference, calf circumference and triceps skinfold thickness. Weight was measured to the nearest 0.1 kg using a weigh chair (type Arjo CFA 2000). Knee height was measured in a sitting position. Bedridden residents were measured in a supine position. Knee and ankle had to be bent at 90°. Knee height was recorded to the nearest 0.1 cm for all participants, using a knee height sliding caliper provided by the Austrian Society for Clinical Nutrition (AKE). Body height was calculated from knee height using the following equations for white non-Hispanic subjects above age 60 [26,27]:

male: 78.31 + (1.94 x knee height [cm]) – (0.14 x age [y])

female: 82.21 + (1.85 x knee height [cm]) – (0.21 x age [y])

The Body Mass Index (BMI) was calculated from body weight (kg) divided by body height squared (m²). BMI was stratified for three groups. A BMI less than 20 kg/m² was considered as low, within 20 and 30 kg/m² as normal, above 30 kg/m² as obese and greater than or equal to 35 kg/m² as severely obese.

Measurements of mid-arm circumference (MAC), waist circumference (WC) and calf circumference (CC) were carried out with a flexible measuring tape and were recorded to the nearest 0.1 cm. Mid-arm circumference was measured on the left side at the mid-point between the tip of the shoulder and the tip of the elbow between olecranon process and acromion. Triceps skinfold thickness (TSF) was measured at the same position with a GPM skinfold caliper to the nearest 0.2 mm (DKSH Switzerland Ltd.). Waist circumference was measured at a level midway between the lower rib margin and iliac crest with the tape all around the body in horizontal position. Calf circumference was measured in a supine or sitting position on the left side at the widest point without compressing the subcutaneous tissue. The mean value from two consecutive measurements was recorded for all parameters.

Functional parameters

Measurement of handgrip strength (HGS) was carried out using a Vigorimeter (by Martin, Germany), recording to the nearest 0.2 kPa. For the timed 'up and go' test (TUG), the residents were asked to stand up from an armchair, to walk three meters, turn around, return to the chair and sit down again. The time needed was measured to the nearest one second. The Index of Activities of Daily Living (ADL) according to Barthel [28] was recorded by the nursing staff. Residents with a score between 65 and 100 points were considered as being independent, residents with a score between 35 and 60 points needed assistance and residents who reached a score <35 points required a high level of care.

All measurements and questionnaires were completed at baseline (t0) and repeated after twelve months (t12). Mortality data were collected from the residents' medical records.

Statistics

Statistical analysis was performed using SPSS© version 17.0 (SPSS for Windows, SPSS Inc., Chicago, IL, USA) and SAS (version 9.1, SAS Institute, Cary, NC, USA). Results are given in mean ± standard deviation (SD) in normally distributed data. The correlations among continuous variables were assessed using Spearman's Rho correlation coefficient. T-tests for independent and dependent samples, respectively, were used to compare differences in variables between baseline and follow-up, in case of normally distributed data. ANOVA was used for statistical comparisons of the distribution of functional parameters between different BMI groups. To analyze the association of BMI and the different functional parameters, respectively, with mortality risk, a Cox proportional hazard model was used, adjusted for the potentially confounding factors age and gender. Statistical tests were performed two-sided. A p-value <0.05 was regarded as significant. In view of the exploratory nature of the analyses, no alpha adjustment techniques were employed.

Results

Study population

From 322 potentially eligible residents, 10 residents under the age of 65 years (8.2%) and 10 residents (8.2%) in palliative care were excluded. 102 residents were not included in the present study for the following reasons: 28 residents did not wish to participate in the study (23.0% of non-participating residents). The legal proxies of 42 residents did not agree to their participation in the study (34.4%). Proxies were inaccessible in another 14 cases (11.5%). 4 residents (3.3%) did not participate due to acute hospitalization, 3 (2.5%) were infected with multi-resistant bacterial strains and 2 (1.6%) residents moved to other institutions. For 9 (7.4%) residents other reasons led to their non-participation. The mean age of the non-participating residents (82.8±11.5 years) was significantly lower than that of the participating residents.

147 female and 53 male residents were included (mean age 85.5±7.8 years). All participants were white. Women were significantly older than men (p<0.05). The MMSE was applicable to 91.0% of the residents. 75.5% of these showed results indicating relevant cognitive impairment (<24 points). The GDS was completed in 71.0% of the residents. 50.0% of these were found to have a score indicative of overt depression (at least 5 points). With regard to the ADL, 28.0% of the residents were categorized as independent, 29.5% needed assistance and 42.5% required a high level of care. Baseline characteristics of the study population stratified for BMI groups are shown in table XIII.

Table XIII: Characteristics at baseline

BMI groups	< 20	n	20 - 30	n	> 30	n	p-value†	r_s with BMI‡
Age [y]	88.5 ± 6.3	17	85.9 ± 7.5	136	83.3 ± 8.8	47	0.039	-0.111*
MMSE [points/30]	12.9 ± 10.7	15	14.4 ± 10.7	124	21.0 ± 8.8	44	0.001	0.194*
TSF [mm]	10.5 ± 3.8	17	16.2 ± 5.4	136	24.0 ± 5.6	47	0.000	0.738*
WC [cm]	83.6 ± 7.9	17	93.6 ± 10.7	136	112.6 ± 9.2	47	0.000	0.803*
MAC [cm]	22.1 ± 1.9	17	27.4 ± 2.9	136	33.9 ± 3.3	47	0.000	0.873*
CC [cm]	27.4 ± 2.8	17	31.7 ± 3.9	136	37.5 ± 5.0	47	0.000	0.694*
HGS [kPa]	25.8 ± 18.2	13	36.3 ± 18.0	107	46.8 ± 17.4	44	0.000	0.327*
MNA score	15.7 ± 4.2	17	20.8 ± 3.6	125	23.4 ± 3.1	46	0.000	0.429*
drugs [n]	7.5 ± 4.8	17	7.8 ± 5.9	136	7.8 ± 4.5	47	0.964	0.086
GDS [points/15]	5.2 ± 4.0	10	5.7 ± 3.6	94	4.4 ± 3.2	38	0.148	-0.150
TUG [sec]	27.8 ± 14.2	4	29.7 ± 18.1	55	25.5 ± 15.7	26	0.541	0.046
ADL	31.2 ± 28.0	17	40.4 ± 28.2	136	49.5 ± 28.2	47	0.045	0.138

†tested with ANOVA, ‡Spearman's Rho correlation coefficient, BMI Body Mass Index, GDS Geriatric Depression Scale, MMSE Mini Mental State Examination, TSF triceps skinfold thickness, WC waist circumference, MAC mid-arm circumference, CC calf circumference, HGS handgrip strength, TUG timed "up and go", ADL Barthel's Activities of Daily Living, MNA Mini Nutritional Assessment

Nutritional status and functional parameters at baseline

The prevalence of low BMI was 8.5% and of normal BMI 68.0%. Obesity was present in 17.5%, severe obesity in 6% (total with BMI >30: 23.5%). Baseline data on age, anthropometric measurements (TSF, WC, MAC, CC), functional parameters (HGS, TUG, ADL) and nutritional screening (MNA) stratified for BMI categories are presented in table XIII.

While recent weight loss above 5% of body weight within the three months before study inclusion was present more often in those with low BMI, it only affected 11.8% of this group. On the contrary 35.3% of residents in the lowest BMI group, 52.6% with normal BMI and 66% with high BMI group had gained weight during this period.

HGS and ADL score was highest and the time needed to perform the TUG was lowest in the high BMI group. The lowest BMI group consistently had the lowest values for functional parameters (p<0.05), except for the TUG. A weak negative correlation was found for BMI and age, while moderately strong and strong positive correlations were calculated for BMI and anthropometric values. With regard to the functional parameters, a positive correlation was shown for BMI and HGS. No correlation with BMI was found for the TUG and ADL score.

Comorbidity

The most prevalent chronic diseases in this age group were recorded at baseline. The high BMI group suffered more often from diabetes mellitus type 2, hypertension, congestive heart failure, hyperthyroidism, hypothyroidism and osteoarthritis than residents with low or normal BMI (figure III), while the number of drugs taken daily differed insignificantly between the three BMI groups (low BMI: 4.8 ± 3.0, normal BMI: 5.5 ± 3.1, high BMI: 5.3 ± 2.3 drugs/d, p-value: 0.701). Significant differences between the BMI groups with regard to their cognitive status, measured by MMSE, were shown, while the depression scale did not demonstrate significant differences.

One-year follow-up

14 participants dropped out during the follow-up due to relocation, withdrawal and hospitalization. 47 deceased during the study period. After the 12 month follow-up, 33.1% of survivors had lost at least 5% weight, 23% were stable and the majority of 43.9% had gained weight.

Parameters of functionality measured at baseline and after follow-up for the surviving group, stratified for BMI categories, are shown in table XV. Data still showed significant differences between BMI groups for HGS at baseline and after one year and for ADL scores after one year. In the group with normal BMI a significant decline of HGS, TUG and ADL was observed, while there was no significant change in those with high BMI and those with low BMI.

The distribution of the BMI of all participants, survivors and deceased, are shown in table XIV. The surviving group showed significantly higher BMI values than the group of the deceased (26.9 vs. 24.3 kg/m², p<0.05).

The lowest mortality rate was observed in the obese (12.8%), with no deaths after 12 months in the severely obese (BMI ≥35 kg/m²; n=12, not shown). Mortality was highest in residents with low BMI (58.8%) (figure VIII).

The different Cox regression analyses, all adjusted for age and gender, yielded the following results:

(i) a significantly increased risk of mortality for the group with low BMI (HR 3.4; 95% CI 1.6-7.0) while obesity was associated with a decreased mortality risk, although this association was not significant (HR 0.5 95% CI 0.2-1.3), considering the normal weight group (BMI 20-30 kg/m²) as a reference

(ii) no significant association between the functional parameters (HGS, TUG, ADL) and mortality.

Figure IX: Prevalence of diseases stratified for BMI groups

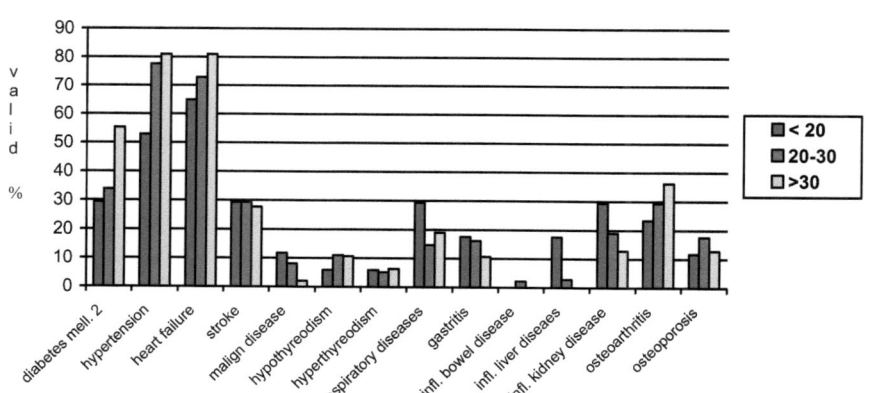

Table XIV: BMI distribution of all participants, deceased and surviving participants

BMI group	< 20	20 – 30	> 30
All [%] n = 200	8.5	68.0	23.5
Survivors [%] n = 139	5.0	68.3	26.6
Deceased [%] n = 47	21.3	66.0	12.8

Figure X: Kaplan-Meier survival estimated by BMI categories

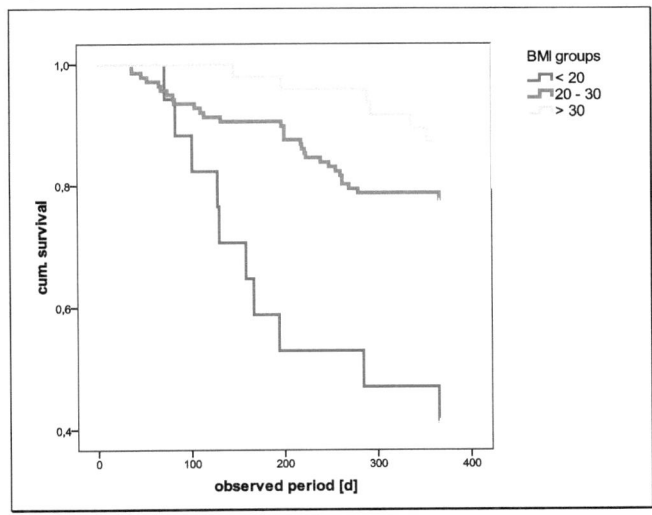

Table XV: Follow-up data of function stratified for BMI groups

BMI groups		< 20			20 - 30			>30			
		n	p-value§		n	p-value§		n	p-value§	p-value†	r_s with BMI‡
number		6			71			33			
HGS [kPa]	t 0	24.5 ± 16.9	0.223	37.2 ± 17.4	71	0.002	47.6 ± 18.5	33	0.275	0.003	0.319*
	t 12	26.5 ± 17.6	6	33.6 ± 18.9	71		45.7 ± 21.7	33		0.008	0.288*
TUG [sec]	t 0	34.5 ± 14.8	2	0.323	23.3 ± 8.2	29	0.007	23.5 ± 9.3	16	0.907	0.226	0.000
	t 12	25.5 ± 7.8	2	30.6 ± 15.3	29		23.8 ± 9.6	16		0.261	0.054
ADL	t 0	42.1 ± 33.1	7	0.649	41.8 ± 27.8	95	0.001	52.0 ± 26.4	37	0.375	0.162	0.118
	t 12	39.3 ± 28.6	7	35.6 ± 29.0	95		53.9 ± 29.3	37		0.006	0.212*

§comparing of the functional development from t0 to t 12, tested with t-test, †comparing of the functionality of the three BMI groups, tested with ANOVA, ‡Spearman's Rho correlation coefficient, *significant (p<0.05), HGS handgrip strength, TUG timed 'up and go', ADL Barthel's Activities of Daily Living

Discussion

While during the past two decades a high prevalence of malnutrition was frequently found in nursing home residents [29,30], the present study showed only a low prevalence of this condition. In contrast, we observed a high prevalence of obesity. In two European studies and one Australian study in nursing home residents the prevalence of obesity was similar to ours, with 22.9%, 21% and 20%, respectively [31-33]. 21% of obese female and 20% of obese male residents were found in German nursing homes [34]. A slightly lower prevalence of 17.8% was found in US nursing home residents [1]. While all of the aforementioned studies were based on the WHO cut-off at 30 kg/m², Grabowski defined obesity as BMI >28 kg/m² and reported a prevalence of 21.4% in the observed population of institutionalized elderly from the US [19]. In contrast, a much lower prevalence of obesity with only 6.3% was found in institutionalized elderly from Venezuela [35]. In the Third National Health and Nutrition Examination Survey (NHANES III) a prevalence of obese elderly (≥30 kg/m²) of 17.4% in men and 21.2% in women was reported among community-dwelling elderly [3]. In homebound US older adults the prevalence was 23% for obese (30-34.9 kg/m²) and 15% for severely obese elderly (≥35 kg/m²) [7]. Based on the above study results it may be stated that in western countries the prevalence of obesity among nursing home residents is similar to its prevalence in community-dwelling elderly and in those that are homebound. The situation seems to be different in emerging nations. Here the characteristics of those that are admitted to nursing homes most probably differ significantly with regard to nutritional status from European countries and the US.

In the present study a BMI less than 20 kg/m² was categorized as low according to the recommendations of the ESPEN guidelines for nutritional screening [36]. We decided to define the BMI range between 20 and 30 kg/m² as normal, as there has been wide agreement that BMI values between 20 and 25 kg/m² are in general considered to be the normal weight range in older individuals while the lowest mortality was shown for older individuals with BMI between 25 and 30 kg/m² [37]. In our view, the overweight category appropriately used in younger individuals therefore had to be questioned for the older population. According to the WHO and the ESPEN criteria, a BMI value above 30 kg/m² was considered to indicate obesity and a BMI ≥ 35 kg/m² was considered as severely obese [36,38].

In the present study, higher BMI was associated with higher cognitive status measured by MMSE. In the scientific literature, data on the association of BMI and the risk of becoming demented are inconsistent [39]. Studies which had also used the MMSE to test cognitive status found an increased risk for incident dementia in underweight (<18.5 kg/m²) as well as in obese (>30 kg/m²) elderly [40]. The association of low BMI with dementia may be interpreted as a consequence of declining BMI during the years preceding the onset of dementia. When considering the association of high BMI with dementia it has been hypothesized that inflammatory and hormonal processes in the adipose tissue may be of special relevance in this context [41]. However, it has to be stressed that the present study may not be directly comparable to the aforementioned scientific papers, as the assessment of cognitive status and the setting of the studies are different.

In the present study, higher BMI values were associated with greater handgrip strength and higher ADL scores at baseline. After one year, functional parameters including handgrip strength, timed 'up and go' and ADL score remained stable in the obese study participants while those with normal BMI showed a decline in this regard. The results of the low BMI group have, however, to be interpreted cautiously. The small number of completed tests may have contributed to those results, as some tests could not be performed as a consequence of immobility and death.

Handgrip strength may be regarded as a suitable test for assessing muscle strength in older individuals in daily routine [42]. However, data on the association of handgrip with BMI are inconsistent. In one study a positive correlation between these two parameters was shown in community-dwelling people [43], while in another study this correlation was not confirmed in women and even a negative correlation was shown in men [44]. Higher BMI, higher percentage of body fat and a greater waist circumference were identified as parameters indicating a higher risk of incident mobility limitations in older well-functioning adults [45]. In studies by Visser and Zamboni, DEXA (Dual energy X-ray absorptiometry) was applied for body composition analysis. It was shown that the percentage of body fat was associated with mobility-related disability and that in women the influence of fat mass was more relevant for functionality than that of fat free mass [46,47]. In addition, fat-free mass was not a significant predictor of mobility-related disability, nor was weight change over a 3-year follow-up [48]. In further studies, the complex relationship between muscle and fat with regard to functionality was also illustrated by the observation that fat infiltration of the mid-thigh muscle was associated with lower strength and that this infiltration constituted an independent risk factor for incident mobility limitations [49,50].

While knowledge on the relationship between obesity and functionality in community-dwelling elderly is steadily growing, there have been very few studies with this focus in nursing home residents.

In the present study, relevant functional deficits were present in all BMI groups. However, they were observed to a larger extent in those with low and normal BMI than in those with high BMI. Nursing home residents represent a highly selected group of older individuals who show severe functional limitations which have led in most cases to their nursing home admission. Therefore the functional background of this population differs significantly from that of community-dwelling older persons. One has to be aware of this specific situation when study results on the relationship between BMI and functionality and on change of functionality over time are interpreted.

One hypothesis to explain this obvious paradoxical observation in nursing home residents suggests that those with low and normal BMI are at higher risk of relevant sarcopenia than those with higher BMI. As sarcopenia is usually a continuous process, the first group will also have a higher risk of a progressive loss of strength and power, which leads to deterioration in more complex functional tasks as well. In this context, it has to be noted that nursing home residents in general show a low level of functionality, being the most relevant reason for their admission in most instances. The described relationship between BMI and functionality therefore applies specifically to the nursing home population and not to independently living older persons.

More research is necessary to clarify these inconsistencies. Unfortunately, DEXA is highly unfeasible in this population and bioimpedance analysis, which may be considered an alternative, shows some serious disadvantages with regard to the reliability of measurements. Here the varying degrees of hydration are of special concern.

Another important observation in this context is that in the nursing home functional deficits seem to be more important in the pathogenesis of malnutrition than acute or chronic comorbidity [51]. As the two groups with low and normal BMI showed higher degrees of functional impairment at baseline (table 2), they might also be considered to be at higher risk of further functional deterioration, which then might be interpreted as a consequence of malnutrition.

In our study, multimorbidity was present in all participants. Although the residents in the highest BMI group showed higher levels of functionality and lower mortality, they suffered more often from chronic, mainly cardiovascular diseases than residents with low or normal BMI. These data support the concept of functionality being more relevant for nutritional status in nursing home residents than chronic comorbidity.

Mortality was lower in those residents with high BMI when compared to those in the low and normal BMI range. Data on the relationship between BMI and mortality for the older population in general still have to be considered as contradictory. Several large-scale studies explored the association between BMI and mortality in older persons [12-16]. In an extensive study of almost 900,000 participants, the lowest mortality has been reported at about BMI 22.5-25 kg/m² [52]. This study did not focus on older persons but included adults with a minimum age of 35 years. These results are comparable to those of a study by Pischon and co-workers. Here the lowest relative risk was shown for a BMI of 23.5 kg/m² in men and 24.3 kg/m² in women aged at least 65 years [53]. Al Snih found the lowest hazard ratios for mortality in elderly above 65 years with a BMI between 25 and 30 kg/m² and, in contrary to our results of nursing home residents, the highest hazards for mortality were reported in older persons with a BMI above 35 kg/m² [37].

Mortality is significantly higher in nursing home residents when compared to the older population in general. In this specific population, higher BMI values may be considered to represent a survival advantage in the sense of energy and somatic protein reserve which will be of value in a time of crisis, the latter being all too frequent in the nursing home population. However, at present it cannot be excluded that higher BMI only indicates a condition where the individual is only at minor risk of losing weight and muscle mass, both of which would indicate an increase in mortality. In the present study, obese subjects showed not only the best survival rate but also better functionality. In this regard, our results are similar to those of a recent study by Gale that observed an inverse relationship between handgrip strength and mortality [54]. The same relationship has also been observed in geriatric patients [55].

The results on functionality and mortality observed in the present study may be seen in the context of phenomena referred to as 'paradoxical epidemiology'. Well-known examples are populations with advanced heart failure, terminal kidney disease, and in some aspects also the aging population [56]. We believe that our population shares some features with these examples, as the nursing home population shows high mortality in general and a high degree of relevant comorbidity and multimedication. For this reason, we believe that nursing home residents may now be regarded as another population that shows relevant features of paradoxical epidemiology.

While it is well-proven that obesity in mid-life has a negative impact on functionality, morbidity and mortality, this may not be true for nursing home residents. In this highly selected population with severely decreased functionality, obesity may be regarded as a protective factor with regard to functionality and mortality.

References IV

1. Lapane KL, Resnik L. Obesity in nursing homes: An escalating problem. J Am Geriatr Soc 2005;53:1386-1391.
2. Bradway C, DiResta J, Fleshner I, Polomano RC. Obesity in Nursing Homes: A Critical Review. J Am Geriatr Soc 2008; 56(8):1528-35.
3. Davison KK, Ford ES, Cogswell ME, Dietz WH. Percentage of Body Fat and Body Mass Index Are Associated with Mobility limitations in People Aged 70 and older from NHANES III. J Am Geriatr Soc 2002;50:1802-1809.
4. Jensen GL, Friedmann JM. Obesity is associated with functional decline in community-dwelling rural older persons. J Am Geriatr Soc 2002;50:918-923.
5. Jenkins KR. Obesity's effects on the onset of functional impairment among older adults. Gerontologist 2004;44(2):206-16.
6. Blaum CS, Xue QL, Michelon E, et al. The Association between Obesity and the Frailty Syndrome in Older Women: the Women's Health and Aging Studies. J Am Geriatr Soc 2005;53:927-934.
7. Sharkey JR, Ory MG, Branch LG. Severe Elder Obesity and 1-Year Diminished Lower Extremity Physical Performance in Homebound Older Adults. J Am Geriatr Soc 2006;54:1407-1413.
8. Elkins JS, Whitmer RA, Sidney S, et al. Midlife Obesity and Long-Term Risk of Nursing Home Admission. Obesity 2006;14:1472-1478.
9. Zizza CA, Herring A, Stevens J, Popkin BM. Obesity Affects Nursing-Care Facility Admission among Whites but Not Blacks. Obes Res 2002;10:816-823.
10. Felix HC. Personal Care Assistance Needs of Obese Elders Entering Nursing Homes. J Am Med Dir Assoc 2008;9(5):319-326.
11. Bales CW and Buhr G. Is obesity bad for older persons? A systematic review of the pros and cons of weight reduction in later life. J Am Med Dir Assoc. 2008;9(5):302-12.
12. Harris T, Cook EF, Garrison R, et al. Body mass index and mortality among non-smoking older persons. The Framingham Heart Study. JAMA 1988;259(10):1520-1524.
13. Cornoni-Huntley JC, Harris TB, Everett DF, et al. An Overview of Body weight of Older Persons, including the impact on mortality. J Clin Epidemiol 1991;44(8):743-753

14. Grabowski DC, Ellis, JE. High Body Mass Index Does Not Predict Mortality in Older People: Analysis of the Longitudinal Study of Aging. J Am Geriatr Soc 2001;49:968-979.
15. DeVore PA. Assessment of nutritional status and obesity in elderly patients as seen in general medical practice. South Med J. 1993;86(9):1008-10.
16. Janssen I. Morbidity and Mortality Risk Associated With an Overweight BMI in Older Men and Women. Obesity 2007;15(7):1827-1840.
17. Beck A-M, Damkjaer K. Optimal Body Mass index in a nursing home population. J Nutr Health Aging 2008;12:1-3.
18. Volpato S, Romagnoni F, Soattin L, et al. Body Mass Index, Body Cell Mass, and 4-Year All-Cause Mortality Risk in Older Nursing Home Residents. J Am Geriatr Soc 2004;52:886–891.
19. Grabowski DC, Campbell CM, Ellis JE. Obesity and mortality in elderly nursing home residents. J Gerontol A Biol Sci Med Sci. 2005;60(9):1184-1189.
20. Folstein MF, Folstein S, McHugh PR: Mini Mental State: a practical method for grading cognitive state of patients for the clinician. J Psychiatr Res 1975;12:189-198
21. Lesher EL and Berryhill JS: Validation of the Geriatric Depression Scale-short form among inpatients. J Clin Psychol 1994;50:256-60.
22. Internet: www.mna-elderly.com 31.01.2009.
23. Guigoz Y, Vellas B, Garry PJ: Mini Nutritional Assessment: a practical assessment tool for grading the nutritional state of elderly patients. Facts Res Gerontol 1994;(2):15-60.
24. Guigoz Y, Vellas B, Garry PJ: Assessing the Nutritional Status of the elderly. The Mini Nutritional Assessment as Part of the Geriatric Evaluation. Nutrition reviews 1996;54:59-65.
25. Bauer JM, Kaiser M, Anthony P, et al. The Mini Nutritional Assessment-Its History, Today's Practice, and Future Perspectives. Nutr Clin Pract 2008;23(4):388-96.
26. Chumlea W, Roche A, Steinbaugh M: estimating stature from knee height for persons 60-90 years of age. J Am Geriatr Soc 1985;33:116-120.
27. Chumlea WW, Guo S, Wholihan K, et al. Stature predictions equations for elderly non-Hispanic white, non-Hispanic black and Mexican American persons developed from NHANES-III data. J Amer dietet Assoc 1998;98:137-142.

28. Mahoney FI and Barthel DW: Functional Evaluation: The Barthel Index. Maryland State Medical Journal 1965;14: 61-65.
29. Silver AJ, Morley JE, Strome LS, et al. Nutritional status in an academic nursing home. J Am Geriatr Soc 1988;36:487-491.
30. Thomas DR, Verdery RB, Gardner L, et al. A prospective study of outcome from protein-energy malnutrition in nursing home residents. J Parenter Enteral Nutr 1991;15: 400-404.
31. Cairella G, Baglio G, Censi L, et al. Mini Nutritional Assessment (MNA) and nutritional risk in elderly. A proposal of nutritional surveillance system for the Department of Public Health. Ann Ig. 2005;17(1):35-46.
32. Abajo del Alamo C, García Rodicio S, Calabozo Freile B, et al. A protocol of assessment, follow-up and nutritional action at a nursing home. Nutr Hosp. 2008;23(2):100-4.
33. Grieger J, Nowson C, Ackland ML. Anthropometric and biochemical markers for nutritional risk among residents within an Australian residential care facility. Asia Pac J Clin Nutr. 2007;16(1):178-86.
34. Heseker H, Stehle P, Bai J, et al. Ernährung älterer Menschen in stationären Einrichtungen (ErnSTES-Studie). In: Deutsche Gesellschaft für Ernährung (editor): Ernährungsbericht 2008. Druck Center Meckenheim GmbH, Meckenheim 2008:157-204.
35. Díaz N, Meertens L, Solano L, Peña E. Nutritional characterization by anthropometrics of institutionalized and non-institutionalized elderly Venezuelan. Invest Clin. 2005;46(2):111-9.
36. ESPEN Guidelines for Nutrition Screening 2002. Kondrup J, Allison SP, Elia M, et al. Clin Nutr 2003;22(4):415–421.
37. Al Snih S, Ottenbacher KJ, Markides KS, et al. The Effect of Obesity on Disability vs Mortality in Older Americans. Arch Intern Med. 2007:23;167(8):774-80.
38. World Health Organisation WHO: http://apps.who.int/bmi/index.jsp?introPage=intro_3.html
39. Gustafson D. A life course of adiposity and dementia. Eur J Pharmacol 2008;585(1):163-75.
40. Peters R, Beckett N, Geneva M, et al. Sociodemographic and lifestyle risk factors for incident dementia and cognitive decline in the HYVET._Age Ageing. 2009;38(5):521-7.

41. Gustafson D. Adiposity indices and dementia. Lancet Neurol 2006;5:713-20.
42. Bauer JM, Kaiser MJ, Sieber CC. Sarcopenia in Nursing Home Residents. J Am Med Dir Assoc 2008;9(8):545-551.
43. Schlüssel MM, dos Anjos LA, de Vasconcellos MT, Kac G. Reference values of handgrip dynamometry of healthy adults: a population-based study. Clin Nutr. 2008;27(4):601-7.
44. Luna-Heredia E, Martin-Pena G, Ruiz-Galiana J. Handgrip dynamometry in healthy adults. Clin Nutr 2005;24:250–258.
45. Koster A, Patel KV, Visser M, et al. Joint Effects of Adiposity and Physical Activity on Incident Mobility Limitaions in Older Adults. J Am Geriatr Soc 2008;6:636-643.
46. Visser M, Harris T, Langlois J, et al. Body fat and skeletal muscle mass in relation to physical disability in very old men and women of the Framingham Heart Study. L Gerontol A Biol Sci Med Sci 1998;53A:M214-221.
47. Zamboni M, Turcato E, Santana H, et al. The relationship between body composition and physical performance in older women. J Am Geriatr Soc 1999;47:1403-1408.
48. Visser M, Langlois J, Guralnik JM, et al. High body fatness, but not low fat-free mass, predicts disability in older men and women: the Cardiovascular Health Study. Am L Clin Nutr 1998;68:584-590.
49. Goodpaster BH, Carlson CL, Visser M, et al.. The association between skeletal muscle composition and strength in the elderly: the Health ABC study. J Appl Physiol. 2001;90:2157-2165.
50. Visser M, Goodpaster BH, Kritchevsky SB, et al. Muscle Mass, Muscle Strength, and Muscle Fat Infiltration as Predictors of Incident mobility Limitations in Well-Functioning Older Persons. J Gerontol 2005;60(3):324-333.
51. Romagnoni F, Zuliani G, Bollini C, et al. Disability is associated with malnutrition in institutionalized elderly people. The I.R.A. Study. Istituto di Riposo per Anziani. Aging (Milano) 1999;11(3):194-9.
52. Prospective Studies Collaboration. Body-mass index and cause-specific mortality in 900 000 adults: collaborative analysis of 57 prospective studies. Lancet 2009;373(9669):1083-1096.
53. Pischon T, Boeing H, Hoffmann K, Bergmann M. General and Abdominal Adiposity and Risk of Death in Europe. N Engl J Med 2008;359:2105-2.

54. Gale CR, Martyn CN, Cooper C, Sayer AA. Grip strength, body composition, and mortality. Int J Epidemiol. 2007;36(1):228-35.
55. Philips P. Grip strength, mental performance and nutritional status as indicators of mortality risk among female geriatric patients. Age Aging 1986;15:53-56.
56. Kalantar-Zadeh K, Horwich TB, Oreopoulos A, Kovesdy CP, Younessi H, Anker SD, Morley JE. Risk factor paradox in wasting diseases. Curr Opin Clin Nutr Metab Care. 2007;10(4):433-42.

CHAPTER FIVE

General Discussion

The nutritional situation of elderly people influences their quality of life, as it is closely associated with functionality, morbidity and mortality (KWON ET AL. 2007, BISCHOFF-FERRARI ET AL. 2004, VOLPATO ET AL. 2004, DE GROOT AND VAN STAVEREN 2002, AMARANTOS ET AL. 2001). Cognitive and physical deficits lead to an increased risk of an insufficient nutritional status, which is highly prevalent in elderly people and therefore concerns nursing home residents in particular. Consequently, malnutrition particularly appears in the elderly population, which has already been shown in several studies and reviews (GASKILL ET AL. 2008, SALVI ET AL. 2008, PAULY ET AL. 2007, PIRLICH ET AL. 2006). Nevertheless, a gold standard for the identification of malnutrition or the risk for malnutrition is still lacking.

The focus of this thesis was the analysis of different methods for the assessment of the nutritional situation of nursing home residents, the monitoring for a one-year follow-up period and, finally, the examination of associations between nutritional status, functionality and mortality in this setting. To my knowledge, this is the first longitudinal study, which investigated the aforementioned parameters in the population of nursing home residents.

Chapter two aimed at the comparison of two different methods for the application of the Mini Nutritional Assessment (MNA), a screening tool, which was recommended for the identification of malnutrition or its risk in frail elderly people (KONDRUP ET AL. 2003, GUIGOZ ET AL. 1996 & 1994). Unfortunately, cognitive deficits, which are highly prevalent in nursing home residents, were not considered when the tool was developed. Consequently, elderly people with cognitive deficits were excluded from data collection in many studies or the assessment was completed by nursing staff and/or closed relatives instead without any further description of the methods.

In the present study, the results of MNA, completed by interview with the residents themselves were compared with those, assessed by nursing staff. The comparison of the two approaches showed a lower applicability rate for the residents' interviews than for the estimation by nursing staff, due to the high prevalence of cognitive impaired residents (69% vs. 94%). Agreement of the results of both methods turned out to be low, but improved when cognitive impaired residents were excluded from the analysis. In a further step, the predictive value of the MNA categories with regard to six-month mortality was analyzed. The relationship was statistically stronger when nursing staff completed the MNA. Additionally, the prevalence of mortality among residents who could not complete the MNA was high (44% of deceased residents). This fact emphasizes the importance of nutritional screening in cognitive impaired elderly to assure an early therapeutic nutritional intervention. These insights gained in chapter two lead to the recommendation that MNA in the nursing home setting should be completed routinely by the nursing staff, because the established methods for completion are not comparable, as shown in the present study. The results achieved are reliable, solely by applying the recommended method.

The nutritional situation with regard to specific nutrient blood markers was analyzed in chapter three of the present thesis. This chapter additionally aimed at investigating the associations between nutrient blood level and functionality and mortality. Longitudinal data in this regard are scarce. Most studies which observed the blood status within a follow-up period in nursing home residents, focused on interventional approaches (MOREIRA-PFRIMER ET AL. 2009, BROE ET AL. 2007, LIU ET AL. 2007, WOUTERS-WESSELING ET AL. 2002).

In the present study, mean blood levels of all analyzed parameters were adequate, except from vitamin D. The highest prevalence of low levels below defined cut-off values were observed for vitamin D, albumin and retinol.

The high prevalence of vitamin D deficiency in people worldwide was already investigated in several studies and concerns especially elderly people due to the decreased synthesis in the aged skin (GRANT AND HOLICK 2005) and the high prevalence of immobility and therefore decreased exposure to UV-light. The present nursing home residents were characterized by low physical function and high prevalence of immobility which led to the high prevalence of vitamin D deficiency.

Albumin, ß-carotene, vitamin B_{12} and folate levels in the present nursing home residents were generally comparable to the literature. α-tocopherole was similar to results of community-dwelling elderly and adults.

In the literature, nursing home residents showed generally lower nutrient levels than elderly in the community, if living independently. Comparable results of home-living handicapped elderly are not available yet; further research is required in this setting.

The low prevalence of low α-tocopherol level in blood in the present study refers to a balanced diet with sufficient amount of vegetable oils. Due to the lack of observing the nutritional intake in the present study, no further statement in the regard can be given as well.

A good nutritional status in elderly people contributes to preservation of muscle mass, obviation of sarcopenia and therefore enables a higher functional ability (BARTALI ET AL. 2008 & 2006). In the present residents, retinol, folate and albumin levels showed positive association with functional parameters and thereby confirm these assumptions.

With exception of vitamin D, no differences could be shown between the prevalence of nutrient deficiencies in survivors and deceased in the present study. Vitamin D was positively associated with cumulative one-year survival when differentiated for vitamin D categories. While residents with vitamin D level between 25-50 nmol/l, showed highest mortality, the lowest mortality was found in residents with optimal level of $\geq$75 nmol/l.

Tube-fed residents showed significantly higher levels of vitamin D and folate, lower cholesterol levels, as well as higher α-tocopherol/cholesterol ratios than non tube-fed. This may on the one hand be explained by the higher concentration of most nutrients, vitamins and minerals in artificial food in general and, on the other hand, by the low nutritional intake in physiologic or cognitive disabled elderly who need assistance during eating (SCHMID ET AL. 2003).

For an adequate supply of nutrients in nursing home residents, a well-balanced amount of food, rich in fresh fruit, vegetables and wholemeal products is required. Additionally, a considerable amount of awareness and patience on the part of the nursing staff needed in order to feed residents or support them adequate during their nutritional intake.

It can be concluded that the population of nursing home residents obviously show a high risk of low nutrient blood levels with regard to vitamin D, albumin and retinol. The supply of the other analyzed nutrients, ß-carotene, vitamin B_{12}, folate and α-tocopherol seems to be adequate, indicated by very low deficiency prevalence rates.

As food intake was not assessed in the present study, no conclusions can be drawn about possible associations of the blood levels of the analyzed nutrients and nutritional intake.

In addition to the high prevalence of malnutrition in the elderly, the problem of obesity has been growing in recent decades (LAPANE ET AL. 2005) and concerns both younger independent adults and nursing home residents.

A negative association between body weight and functionality was already investigated in the community (BLAUM ET AL. 2005, DAVISON ET AL. 2002, JENSEN AND FRIEDMANN 2002).

Aim of chapter four was to analyze the association between BMI, functional parameters and mortality. Obesity was defined as BMI above 30 kg/m^2. Analysis revealed that obese residents showed the highest values of functionality, and, regarding the follow-up data, a steady state of functional ability, while residents in the normal BMI range (20-30 kg/m^2) show a decrease of physical functioning within one year. Due to the low number of residents within the low BMI range (<20 kg/m^2) who were able to accomplish the functional tests, the results of this group have to be considered with caution.

However, data also indicate that relevant functional deficits are existing in all BMI groups in the present study, even though residents with low and normal BMI had greater deficits than those with high BMI. These highly relevant functional limitations may have in most cases led in first place to the nursing home admission.

The association between BMI and survival in the present study was unequivocal, as the lowest mortality was found in severe obese residents (BMI >35 kg/m^2). These results contribute to the assumption that higher BMI values represent a functional and survival advantage in this special setting. This might be explained by higher energy and protein reserves with protective properties in time of crisis. In summary, even though it is well-known that obesity in younger and community-dwelling elderly is associated with lower functional ability (KOSTER ET AL. 2008, VISSER ET AL 1998), this fact seems to be no longer true for this nursing home setting, which shows relevant features of paradoxical epidemiology.

References V

AMARANTOS E, MARTINEZ A, DWYER J. Nutrition and Quality of Life in Older Adults. *J Gerontol. 2001,56A:54-64.*

BARTALI B, FRONGILLO EA, GURALNIK JM, STIPANUK MH, ALLORE HG, CHERUBINI A, BANDINELLI S, FERRUCCI L, GILL TM. Serum Concentrations and Decline in Physical Function Among Older Persons. *J Am Med Assoc. 2008;23:308-315.*

BARTALI B, FRONGILLO EA, BANDINELLI S, Lauretani F, Semba RD, Fried LP, Ferrucci L. Low nutrient intake is an essential component of frailty in older persons. *J Gerontol Med Sci. 2006;61A, 589–593.*

BISCHOFF-FERRARI HA, DIETRICH T, ORAV EJ, HU FB, ZHANG Y, KARLSON EW, DAWSON HUGHES B. Higher 25-hydroxyvitamin D concentrations are associated with better lower-extremity function in both active and inactive persons aged $\geq$ 60 y. *Am J Clin Nutr. 2004;80:752-8.*

BLAUM CS, XUE QL, MICHELON E, SEMBA RD, FRIED LP. The Association between Obesity and the Frailty Syndrome in Older Women: the Women's Health and Aging Studies. *J Am Geriatr Soc 2005;53:927-934.*

BROE KE, CHEN TC, WEINBERG J, BISCHOFF-FERRARI HA, HOLICK MF, KIEL DP. A Higher Dose of Vitamin D Reduces the Risk of Falls in Nursing Home Residents: A randomized, Multiple-Dose Study. *J Am Geriatr Soc. 2007;55:234-239.*

DAVISON KK, FORD ES, COGSWELL ME, DIETZ WH. Percentage of Body Fat and Body Mass Index Are Associated with Mobility limitations in People Aged 70 and older from NHANES III. *J Am Geriatr Soc. 2002;50:1802-1809.*

DE GROOT CPGM, VAN STAVEREN WA. Undernutrition in the European SENECA studies. *Clin Geriatr Med. 2002; 18: 699-708.*

GASKILL D, BLACK LJ, ISENRING EA, HASSALL S, SANDERS F, BAUER JD. Malnutrition prevalence and nutrition issues in residential aged care facilities. *Australas J Ageing. 2008;27(4):189-94.*

GRANT WB, HOLICK MF: Benefits and Requirements of Vitamin D for Optimal Health: A Review. *Altern Med Rev. 2005;10(2):94-111.*

GUIGOZ Y, VELLAS B, GARRY PJ: Mini Nutritional Assessment: a practical assessment tool for grading the nutritional state of elderly patients. *Facts Res Gerontol. 1994;(2):15-60.*

GUIGOZ Y, VELLAS B, GARRY PJ. Assessing the Nutritional Status of the elderly. The Mini Nutritional Assessment as Part of the Geriatric Evaluation. *Nutr Rev. 1996; 54: 59-65.*

JENSEN GL, FRIEDMANN JM. Obesity is associated with functional decline in community-dwelling rural older persons. *J Am Geriatr Soc. 2002;50:918-923.*

KONDRUP J, RASMUSSEN HH, HAMBERG O, STANG Z, AND AD HOC ESPEN WORKING GROUP. Nutritional Risk Screening (NRS 2002): a new method based on an analysis of controlled clinical trials. *Clin Nutr. 2003; 22: 321-336.*

KOSTER A, PATEL KV, VISSER M, VAN EIJK JT, KANAYA AM, DE REKENEIRE N, NEWMAN AB, TYLAVSKY FA, KRITCHEVSKY SB, HARRIS TB. Health, Aging and Body Composition Study. Joint Effects of Adiposity and Physical Activity on Incident Mobility Limitaions in Older Adults. *J Am Geriatr Soc. 2008;6:636-643.*

KWON J, SUZUKI T, KIM H, YISHIDA Y, IWASA H. Concomitant lower serum albumin and vitamin D levels are associated with decreased objective physical performance among Japanese community-dwelling elderly. *Gerontol. 2007;53:322-328.*

LAPANE KL, RESNIK L. Obesity in nursing homes: An escalating problem. *J Am Geriatr Soc. 2005;53:1386-1391.*

LIU BA, MCGEER A, MCARTHUR MA, SIMOR AE, AGHDASSI E, DAVIS L, ALLARD JP. Effect of Multivitamin and Mineral Supplementation on Episodes of Infection in Nursing Home Residents: A Randomized, Placebo-Controlled Study. *J Am Ger Soc. 2007;55:35-42.*

MOREIRA-PFRIMER LDF, PEDROSA MAC, TEIXEIRA L, LAZARETTI-CASTRO M. Treatment of Vitamin D Deficiency Increases Lower Limb Muscle Strength in Institutionalized Older People Independently of Regular Physical Activity: A Randomized Double-Blind Controlled Trial. *Ann Nutr Metab. 2009;54:291-300.*

PAULY L, STEHLE P, VOLKERT D. Nutritional situation of elderly nursing home residents. *Z Gerontol Geriatr. 2007;40:3–12.*

PIRLICH M, SCHÜTZ T, NORMAN K, GASTELL S, LÜBKE HJ, BISCHOFF SC, BOLDER U, FRIELING T, GÜLDENZOPH H, HAHN K, JAUCH KW, SCHINDLER K, STEIN J, VOLKERT D, WEIMANN A, WERNER H, WOLF C, ZÜRCHER G, BAUER P, LOCHS H. The German hospital malnutrition study. *Clin Nutr. 2006;25(4):563-72.*

SALVI F, GIORGI R, GRILLI A, MORICHI V, ESPINOSA E, SPAZZAFUMO L, MARINOZZI ML, DESSÌ-FULGHERI P. Mini Nutritional Assessment (short form) and functional decline in older patients admitted to an acute medical ward. *Aging Clin Exp Res. 2008;20(4):322-8*

SCHMID A, WEISS M, HESEKER H. Recording the nutrient intake of nursing home residents by food weighing method and measuring the physical activity. *J Nutr Health Aging 2003;7(5):294-5.*

VISSER M, HARRIS T, LANGLOIS J, HANNAN MT, ROUBENOFF R, FELSON DT, WILSON PW, KIEL DP. Body fat and skeletal muscle mass in relation to physical disability in very old men and women of the Framingham Heart Study. *Gerontol A Biol Sci Med Sci. 1998;53A:M214-221.*

VOLPATO S, ROMAGNONI F, SOATTIN L, BLÈ A, LEOCI V, BOLLINI, C, FELLIN R, ZULIANI G. Body Mass Index, Body Cell mass, and 4-Year All-Cause Mortality Risk in Older Nursing Home Residents. *J Am Geriatr Soc. 2004;52:886-891.*

WOUTERS-WESSELING W, WOUTERS AEJ, KLEIJER CN, BINDELS JG, DE GROOT CPGM, VAN STAVEREN WA. Study of the effect of a liquid nutrition supplement on the nutritional status of psycho-geriatric nursing home patients. *Eur J Clin Nutr. 2002;56:245-251.*

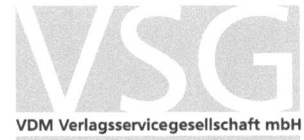
VDM Verlagsservicegesellschaft mbH

Die VDM Verlagsservicegesellschaft sucht für wissenschaftliche Verlage abgeschlossene und herausragende

Dissertationen, Habilitationen, Diplomarbeiten, Master Theses, Magisterarbeiten usw.

für die kostenlose Publikation als Fachbuch.

Sie verfügen über eine Arbeit, die hohen inhaltlichen und formalen Ansprüchen genügt, und haben Interesse an einer honorarvergüteten Publikation?

Dann senden Sie bitte erste Informationen über sich und Ihre Arbeit per Email an *info@vdm-vsg.de*.

Sie erhalten kurzfristig unser Feedback!

VDM Verlagsservicegesellschaft mbH
Dudweiler Landstr. 99
D - 66123 Saarbrücken
Telefon +49 681 3720 174
Fax +49 681 3720 1749
www.vdm-vsg.de

Die VDM Verlagsservicegesellschaft mbH vertritt

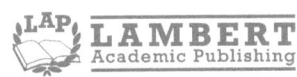
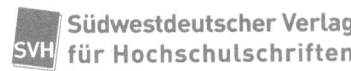

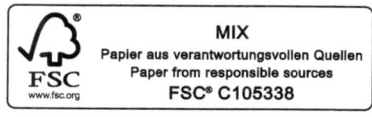

Printed by Books on Demand GmbH, Norderstedt / Germany